BADGES OF MOTHERHOOD

One Mother's Story about Family, Down syndrome, Hospitals, & Faith

By: Evana Sandusky

Written by: Evana Sandusky
Edited by Kim Burger

This is a work of nonfiction. Some names, characters, places, and incidents are changed to protect the identity of other people involved.

Evana Sandusky
Visit my website at http://specialpurposedlife.blogspot.com/

Printed in the United States of America
ISBN: 978-1-7267-3419-6

By: Evana Sandusky

TABLE OF CONTENTS

INTRODUCTION

The signs are all there: you get less sleep, your day is centered around a tiny version of yourself, and you look forward to Mother's Day. Yes, you are a mother. Maybe motherhood has been everything you have dreamed about. Maybe it was nothing like you thought it would be. Still, you find yourself in this unique, yet timeless, role of a mother.

Motherhood has only one requirement: to have a child. That child may have come through natural means, adoption, or marriage. No matter how the child became yours, a new world has come to you that you may have otherwise not have known so intimately.

Once a woman has entered motherhood, she begins learning new skills and having new life experiences, which are referred to as "badges" in this book. These badges tell the story of the achievements and challenges of the mom and her child's care. The badges are symbolic of particularly special times in the mother-child relationship. Some of these badges are kept throughout a mother's life, no matter how much time passes. Other badges can be discarded or lost.

There are some badges that all moms will go through like the Delivery Badge. There are some badges that only some moms will receive, such as the Diagnosis Badge. Some badges are highly anticipated (i.e. Child Baptism Badge) while others are not (i.e. Hospital Care Badge). Some badges can be earned multiple times for separate events or for each child, but some badges are earned only once in a mother's life.

In all, the badges represent triumphs in the mother's life, hardships that have been overcome, skills that were necessary for those moments, and the basic journey of a mom raising her child.

Since 2006, I have been acquiring several badges while parenting my two children. I had no idea just how much my life would change when I became a mother. Parenting has provided the most fulfilling, beautiful, and challenging moments of my life. I hope you enjoy reading about some of my badges and can value the badges you have earned in your journey as well.

By: Evana Sandusky

CHAPTER 1:

THE DELIVERY BADGE

Delivery Badge: This badge is earned when a mother receives her child. While the process may occur through natural means, adoption, or marriage, every mom has a moment when her child entered her life. This badge is earned on that date of delivery.

My Delivery Badge Earned: February 2006

Sleep seemed to evade me through most of my pregnancy. That night was no different. I woke up in the middle of the night with what I thought were hunger pains. These pains felt slightly different from the ones I breathed through before crawling into bed at the beginning of my night. The school where I was employed had graciously given me a baby shower at the end of our work day. I carried all sorts of baby paraphernalia from the shower into the baby's nursery where I dropped it with intentions of going through it over the weekend. I thought I had carried something too heavy or had just been on my feet too long, and I really didn't think too much about my pains at any moment.

I fell back asleep watching television, desperately trying to get some rest before work the next day. I had three weeks left to go in this pregnancy. I couldn't wait to see our baby, especially after such a rocky start.

Months ago, I stood in our narrow hallway outside the bathroom door and told my husband of three years the pregnancy test was positive. Jason was so stunned; he didn't know what to do. He told me to take another test. If it was positive too, then we would talk about the reality of what was happening.

Before we were married, Jason and I had dated for five years, starting in high school. I knew this man, and I knew he needed more proof of this pregnancy. Like a good wife, I provided him with the further evidence that he needed. After that, he agreed I must have been pregnant.

Before we had let anyone else in on our secret, I started spotting. It made me nervous. I didn't know what to do. I called my mom, told her I was pregnant, and immediately followed the good news with the worry that I was having a miscarriage. There was no cute reveal to our family that most couples experience. A frantic phone call was how our immediate family found out we were pregnant.

The visit to the emergency room with my husband and my mother was upsetting. I wasn't given many answers. Maybe I would remain pregnant and maybe I wouldn't—that was all the information I knew when I left the emergency room. It wasn't reassuring. I left there knowing I was still pregnant, at that moment.

The spotting went on for several weeks and I wondered the entire time if I was still pregnant. By then, people had heard we were expecting, and the congratulations started. I didn't know if I should allow myself to be happy yet or not, especially since I was still in the first trimester.

I hadn't planned on being pregnant at that moment, but I wanted the baby from the first second I knew of its existence. I prayed like a desperate woman for the baby to be fine. By the end of the first trimester, the spotting stopped but the pregnancy sickness that started around 8 weeks continued. I had the pleasure of all-day morning sickness for most of my pregnancy. Even though I felt horrible, I was strengthened by the fact that the sickness would have an ending when the baby arrived.

Everything indicated a healthy baby would soon be ours. The grainy black and white images in the ultrasounds left much to the imagination, but I was told everything was developing on track. I declined any prenatal testing that I was offered because I wasn't worried about anything. I was 25 years old and had no family history that would cause concern. Early on, Jason and I just knew we were going to be having a son, but science said differently. Dresses, pink accessories, and hair bows were common gifts after we announced a daughter was coming. We were so excited for her birth in March.

March was not to be her birth month, however. Around 4 am on February 17, 2006, while resting on my couch fighting those hunger pains, my water broke. I naïvely thought this moment would come three weeks later on the baby's due date. The idea of it happening earlier had never occurred to me, which meant I was ill-equipped to leave.

With excitement for what was happening, my husband and I quickly changed and packed for the hospital. As we drove to the hospital, we called our parents and siblings. My brother advised me to stay home for a while, since the baby wouldn't come immediately; our parents echoed the same advice. We didn't listen. We were new to this, so we wanted to see a doctor.

At the hospital, they informed me that my "hunger pains" were contractions. I was well on my way to having this baby and I didn't even know it! Labor came on fast once I arrived in the delivery room. I had decided early on that I would not have an epidural, and fortunately I was able to keep that plan. Instead, I received a medication through an IV, which made me drowsy but helped with the pain. I felt so unprepared for this moment, though I had known for months it was coming. Just a few hours later, at 9 am, the doctor walked in for the grand event. During delivery, the baby's heart rate dropped, and the doctor gave me the impression things needed to move faster. Through a vacuum assist, Jaycee swiftly came into this world.

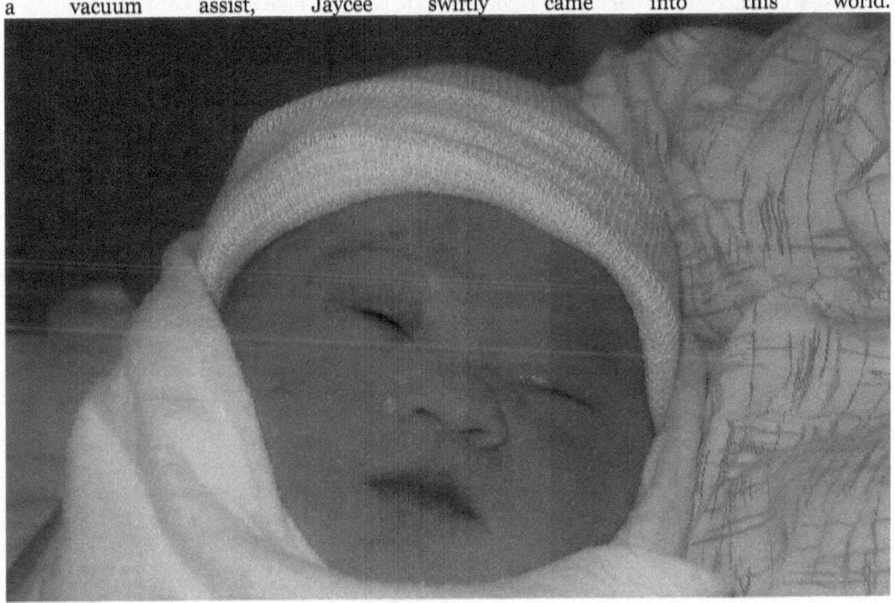

Jaycee at Birth

By: Evana Sandusky

I did a quick glance at this baby that I had been trying to picture for the past several months. Ten toes, ten fingers, two ears, two eyes—everything seemed right. Her cry was weak but present. I knew from television that a cry was a good thing. Her facial features seemed soft and gentle, though very swollen from the delivery. I didn't notice anything out of the ordinary. She was beautiful. It was a surreal moment.

Jaycee was here. She was our first child and my in-laws first grandchild. Everything seemed perfect. I was awarded my first badge—Delivery. *I did it!*

Delivery Badge Earned: August 2009

With one Delivery Badge on my sash, I felt more prepared for my next one. This pregnancy started with familiar feelings of nausea and sickness. Fortunately, this time it did not last the entire pregnancy. The pregnancy overall was less stressful as well, since spotting never occurred. At our 20-week ultrasound, the baby's health all checked out well and I was relieved. Again, we declined any extra prenatal testing because we weren't overly concerned about discovering health issues. We found out that a son would be joining our family. We were beyond happy to welcome another addition.

I knew the due date was not a fixed date to bank on this time. Four weeks before the big day, I was all packed and ready to go, just in case. At the same time, three-year-old Jaycee was scheduled to have her enlarged tonsils and adenoids removed. Even though my last month of pregnancy wasn't a good time to schedule Jaycee's surgery, I decided it would be better to do the procedure before the new baby arrived.

Jaycee's surgery went well but the recovery was horrible. I could not get her to eat or drink. I would beg and plead her to take a sip or a bite of something, anything. I tried giving her a few milliliters of liquid using a syringe. Dehydration concerns prompted a visit to the emergency room for fluids and a stronger pain medication.

Ten days after surgery, the rare complication of this surgery occurred—Jaycee hemorrhaged. I found her in her room shortly after putting her to bed. Her room looked like a crime scene. Blood was everywhere around her and I panicked. Immediately, I started having contractions. We were warned that a hemorrhage could cause death and warranted an immediate trip to the emergency room. As we rushed Jaycee to the closest hospital, thankfully her bleeding stopped.

We were up literally the entire night transporting her from a local hospital to a children's hospital farther away where Jaycee was admitted for observation. When we finally settled into Jaycee's hospital room at 5 am, I was still having contractions. Jason and I were getting nervous at that point. We were two hours from our home where our packed hospital bag sat, and this was no time to have a baby. After having some water and breakfast, my contractions finally stopped.

The next day, Jaycee appeared to be doing well. She was miraculously eating and drinking, so she was discharged. When we got home from our whirlwind adventure, my contractions started again. We were only home for a few hours before we decided to go to the hospital again, but this time it was for me.

At 37 weeks, it was clear I was going to have this baby. I pictured my labor being like my first one, short with a moderate amount of pain. Nevertheless, this labor went on and on. Contractions kept coming and going for over 24 hours. I just wanted it over with after just a few hours of labor. I was exhausted from being in the hospital the day before with Jaycee. I didn't feel like I had any strength to birth this baby. I refused the epidural again, foolishly thinking this labor wouldn't last long. I was wrong, and the pain medications I received did not mask what I was feeling. Finally, the time came. With great effort, I was able to finally see my baby boy for the first time.

My son, Elijah, arrived three weeks early, like his sister. He was my in-laws first grandson and he made Jaycee a big sister. I was ecstatic to receive my second Delivery Badge.

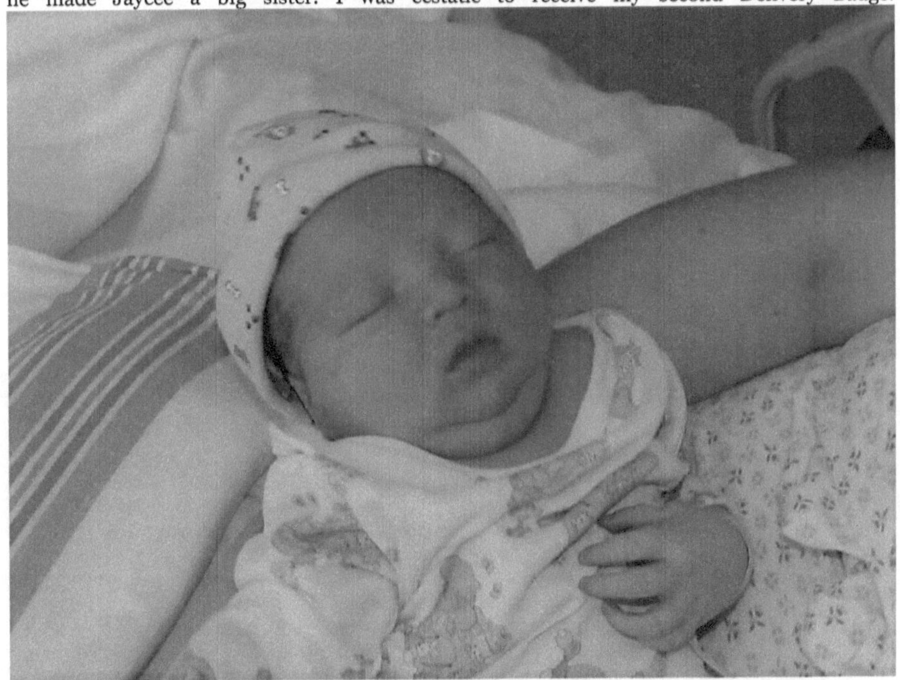

Elijah at Birth

By: Evana Sandusky

CHAPTER 2:

THE DIAGNOSIS BADGE

> *Diagnosis Badge: This badge is earned when a mom is given news that her child has a developmental, educational, or medical diagnosis. Badges are given for a significant diagnosis that requires medical or therapeutic intervention performed by medical or educational specialists. This badge is awarded when a definitive diagnosis is given because the mom's life, as well as the child's, is then changed. Diagnosis badges are sustained as long as the diagnosis remains. Multiple diagnoses badges can be earned.*

Diagnosis Badge Earned: February 18, 2006-Down syndrome

Just hours after her birth, Jaycee was in the nursery being attended to by several staff. We weren't allowed to see her while they were doing whatever it was that they were doing. I thought it odd, but I had no previous experience to really know if it was standard procedure.

Shortly before our separation, I had unsuccessfully tried to nurse Jaycee. During that attempt, her tongue seemed to be stuck to the roof of her mouth. She didn't know what to do, and I didn't know how to get her to nurse. I thought being three weeks early affected her sucking reflex, so I wasn't alarmed at all. Plus, I really didn't feel like I knew what I was doing.

A nurse in the room tried to guide me through the breastfeeding process. After a few minutes of trying, the nurse took Jaycee back to the nursery. I don't remember her excuse for taking her, but she never signaled or stated anything was wrong. Then, we were told lab work need to be completed. Jaycee's body was not keeping her body temperature up, so the doctors wanted her kept in a warm nursery bed. I was concerned but not worried. I suppose the calmness of everyone kept me from being suspicious.

A few hours later though, I had reason to worry. We met Jaycee's pediatrician for the first time after she did her initial assessment. It was hours after delivery when the sweet, female doctor walked into my room. She told me the nurse assisting me in breastfeeding Jaycee noticed my daughter was turning blue during the feed. I was too focused on the task to notice her color change. The doctor then informed me Jaycee was under an oxygen hood. In my mind, oxygen seemed plausible considering she was three weeks early. Perhaps, I would have been worried if she was born right on her due date. I just didn't know.

Then the doctor continued to say she heard a heart murmur. Again, I wasn't too concerned. I did not realize that a heart murmur could mean a heart defect. I suppose the only people I knew who had heart murmurs had innocent ones, not like Jaycee's. This conversation was taking a new direction, but I was optimistic my daughter would be fine.

But then the final piece of information was delivered. The pediatrician said that, based upon her assessment, she was concerned there was a genetic disorder present. The doctor spoke in a caring and compassionate way while she did her best to give my husband and me unforeseen information about our newborn. Still, there's nothing that prepares you emotionally for news you were absolutely never expecting to hear.

I curled up in my hospital bed and cried. My mind immediately went into panic mode. I had a hundred thoughts all at once. What was happening? It wasn't the way I was expecting things to go. My husband practically raced to my bed and immediately started talking to me to calm me down. He assured me things were going to be fine.

As we tried to make sense of what we were just told, our family and friends were on the way to the hospital to celebrate Jaycee's arrival. As family members came in with big smiles, we had to break the news and interrupt the party atmosphere. Upon hearing the news, my father gathered us together and prayed intensely for Jaycee to be fine. I needed people to pray in that moment, but I didn't have the strength to do it. I was in shock, and I was trying to process the news. Prayers began elsewhere as our church was contacted and word spread that something may be wrong with our baby Jaycee.

We soon said good-bye to our daughter as she laid in her incubator prepared to go on her first helicopter ride to a hospital two hours away. Since I didn't get an epidural, I was discharged right after Jaycee left the hospital, so I could be with her. I was thankful the hospital gave me the option to be discharged early. I wouldn't have survived in that room without a baby and with wandering thoughts.

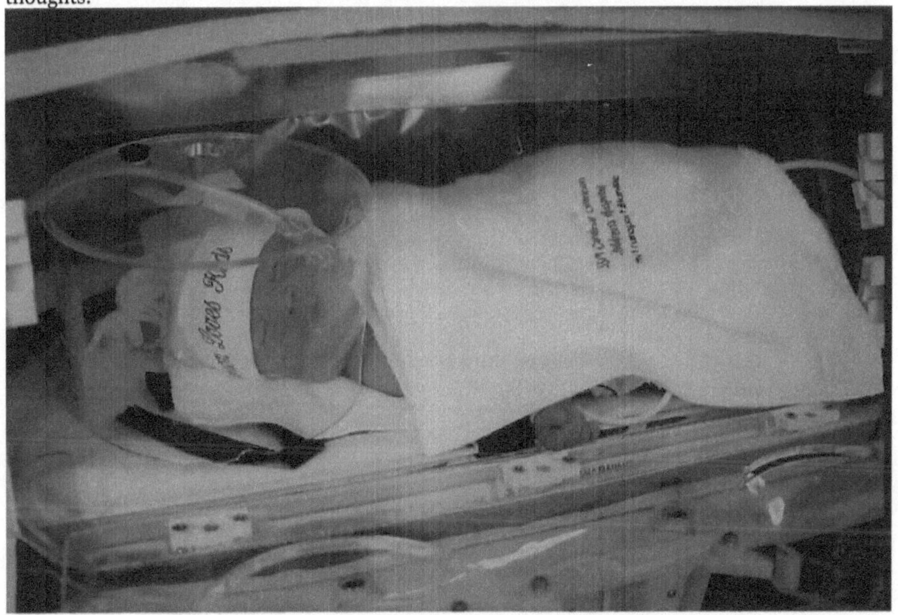

Jaycee Loaded Up for the Helicopter

We had a brief visit with Jaycee that night at her new hospital. She remained on oxygen and had wires and monitors all over her small body. She looked seriously sick. I was afraid to hold her or touch her, not understanding what was going on; I thought I was going to have a healthy baby during my pregnancy.

The neonatal intensive care unit (NICU) was bustling, which made it even more frightening. There were beeps and alarms heard almost constantly, not just from Jaycee but also from the other babies in the room. The lights were extremely bright and the whole place was understandably sterile. Jaycee was being closely monitored by a nurse, but it was too much to process. This wasn't the kind of situation you think you will be in when you have a baby.

The long day of Jaycee's birth turned into a long night. Looking back, I cannot believe I delivered a baby, traveled two hours in a car, and walked around a hospital to see my daughter all

By: Evana Sandusky

on the same day. I suppose I was running on adrenaline. I would pay for all that movement a few days later when my body's pain could no longer be ignored.

At some point, we tried to get some rest in a room offered to us by the hospital. I was glad to have a room to stay in until I found out our sleeping arrangements were bunk beds and a shared bathroom. If you have ever had a baby, you'll understand the downside to these things.

The next morning, we met Jaycee's NICU doctor. He was a small-framed man who clearly had the respect of the other health professionals around him. With our NICU doctor came a handful of doctors in residency and fellowships, as Jaycee was in a teaching hospital. The large group of people surrounded us, and introductions were made. The NICU doctor began his speech, sounding as if he had given it hundreds of times before. He started by pointing to me and said, "If you notice, your baby won't look like your baby pictures." And then he pointed to my husband and said, "She won't look like your baby pictures either. She won't look like either of you because she has Down syndrome."

Those words cut me deep within my soul. It was as if anyone's baby was laying there in front of me rather than my own child. His speech made me feel very disconnected from my child. I was honestly damaged for a couple of years as I wrongly believed my child did not and would not look like me.

As if that wasn't enough, he went on to point out everything "wrong" with Jaycee's body that indicated Down syndrome. She had a straight line across the palm of her hand, extra skin on her neck, low muscle tone (displayed as he flopped her legs around every which way), and a flat nasal bridge. I was warned our baby would have delays in development, an intellectual disability, and may not ever live independently. By the time the discourse ended, I saw only a baby with flaws and problems and was offered little or no positive views. His speech offered no hope, something I needed at the time.

Down syndrome was never on my radar; I was in my 20s after all, and wrongly thought this was ONLY something that happened to older mothers. It was a shock.

So, with a herd of doctors and nurses watching, my first Diagnosis Badge was given to me. I reluctantly took that badge with tears in my eyes and a look of disbelief.

A few days later the genetics test came back. The doctor was correct. Without a doubt, Jaycee had Down syndrome.

At some point in the NICU, we were introduced to people from a Down syndrome support group, but I was not ready to talk or hear anything else. I wish I would have taken that opportunity because I am sure those individuals would have given me the hope and positive outlook I was searching for at that moment. But, I also realize that one's brain and body can only handle so much at one time. I eventually reached out to this group once we were home and settled.

Diagnosis Badge Earned: February 18, 2006-Heart Condition

Right after my husband and I were told Jaycee had Down syndrome, we spent time in the NICU waiting area with our parents and friends who were anticipating news of Jaycee's condition. We discussed Jaycee's Down syndrome and what the doctor had told us. I could barely say anything and mainly cried. Our family was great about encouraging us and offering support. They prayed and let me voice my concerns. When I got the strength to return to my daughter's NICU room an hour or so later, the group of doctors was back with an added member, a cardiologist. I was given a seat off to the side and asked to wait for the cardiology testing to end.

Just as I settled into my chair, a female doctor in training approached me. She essentially started telling me Jaycee's heart had holes in it, blood was mixing, and she would need open-heart surgery. For 9 months, I believed I was going to be a mom to a healthy baby. This doctor's diagnosis was too much for my post pregnancy mind and emotions to handle. Before she could finish her matter-of-fact speech, I was in tears. I made it through the first diagnosis holding back my emotions while the doctor talked, but this time they erupted uncontrollably. Down syndrome was one thing, but a heart condition was much more serious to me. I couldn't process what was happening.

The doctor looked as if I was the first crying parent she had ever encountered. I suppose I could have been, since she was in training. She quietly removed herself without really finishing and retreated to her colleagues still surrounding Jaycee. My husband arrived a few minutes later wondering why in the world I was crying again.

Before I could explain it to Jason, a male doctor cautiously approached us. He re-explained Jaycee's heart problem, drawing a picture to help us understand. She had an atrioventricular heart defect (commonly known as a complete AV canal heart defect). Fundamentally, she had a large hole in the middle of her heart that would lead to pulmonary hypertension, congestive heart failure, and open-heart surgery.

We were asked if we were aware of these problems during the pregnancy. Of course, we weren't, and I don't believe I would have been crying hysterically in front of a small crowd of people if I had known beforehand. In retrospect, the young female doctor who first approached me with this heart diagnosis should have waited for my husband to join me. I also wish she would have presented this bombshell a little more delicately. There's never a good way to deliver bad news, but there are better ways to do it.

There in that NICU room, I received a second Diagnosis Badge for a baby who was just on her second day of life. This Diagnosis Badge came with its own set of problems and life changing issues. Medications were immediately started but wouldn't be needed forever. Before she was two years old, Jaycee would have two open heart surgeries to fully correct her heart problem. One heart surgery was expected, but unfortunately, she needed to have another one to fully fix the leaks in her heart.

My heart, as a mom, hurt for hers. All of it was hard. The diagnosis, the medications, the fears, and the surgery. When you are pregnant with a baby, you never expect to encounter these problems. When they occur, you just have to deal with them. The scariest part about Jaycee's heart diagnosis was knowing her life didn't seem guaranteed, as the heart is a vital organ. I just wanted assurances that her life would be long and productive. A heart diagnosis seemed to take away all those securities other children were provided.

The heart diagnosis was scary for me as a new parent. Little did I know, this was just the beginning.

Diagnosis Badge Earned: 2006/2007-Asthma

When Jaycee was 10 months old, I was still adjusting to the two badges I already received as her mother for different diagnoses. There were so many responsibilities I had caring for a child with developmental delays and heart issues. I was not expecting another badge anytime soon and wasn't sure I could handle another one.

In early winter, Jaycee became sick with a cold, so I took her to see her pediatrician. Her breathing was labored, but I thought her underlying heart issues may be to blame. She coughed and wheezed as the pediatrician listened to her and asked, "Who in your family has asthma?"

My brother has it. My husband had it as a child. But, I never had breathing problems.

She suspected Jaycee had asthma and wanted her to start breathing treatments. I wasn't convinced it was asthma. She tried to give me another Diagnosis Badge that I didn't believe belonged to us. I didn't take it. I thought this was just an isolated incident. I didn't understand asthma or its symptoms. I did do the breathing treatments she prescribed, but I really wasn't sure if they helped.

About five months later, Jaycee was feverish, wheezing, and had labored breathing once again. After a few trips to the doctor's office and treating her at home with breathing treatments for several days, Jaycee was not getting any better. After agonizing over what to do, we decided to take her to the emergency room. As we drove to the hospital, we didn't know if she was really having trouble breathing or if we were overreacting.

At the emergency room, Jaycee was seen right away, and they decided to admit her. Evidently, we weren't overreacting parents. She spent several days on oxygen at a local hospital before being transferred to the nearest children's hospital where she was diagnosed with pneumonia. Finally, I knew her breathing issues were not minor after all. At the children's hospital, several doctors explained to me why Jaycee fit the description for asthma. As much as I didn't want to admit it,

By: Evana Sandusky

Jaycee had another diagnosis. The Diagnosis Badge that I had spent five months contemplating and rejecting now clearly belonged to us, too. I wasn't afraid of asthma at all in the beginning. I thought if I controlled her medications and avoided her triggers that I would be able to manage it—I was so wrong. Her breathing issues, combined with her Down syndrome and heart defect, would make any simple cold anything but simple, which you'll read about in detail later in this book. Add to the fact that Jaycee doesn't have the language skills to verbalize when she's feeling tightness in her chest just exasperates the issue. I have always had to "read" her behaviors and look for signals that something isn't right.

With asthma came nebulizer masks, inhalers, and avoidance of pets, allergens, and any form of smoke. It changed our lifestyle in some ways and at times made me paranoid of flowers, corn fields, any places with hay, and any small accumulations of dust in our house.

I had no idea when Jaycee was diagnosed with asthma just how much it would affect our life in the future. However, her lungs weren't the only body part that needed extra support.

Diagnosis Badge Earned: 2007-Strabismus

"What's wrong with Jaycee's eyes?"

I would ask my husband this question as I studied the out-of-sync eye movements as Jaycee focused on an object when she was a baby. There were also moments when Jaycee's eyes crossed. Usually, it was one eye crossing in though sometimes it was both. At the end of the day or when she was tired, it was worse.

Whenever I worried about Jaycee, I would always consult Jason about my thoughts. I'm not sure if I wanted him to agree with me or tell me I was worrying over nothing. This time he agreed.

Not long after I noticed Jaycee's eyes, I took her for a vision screening when she was under a year old. That led us to being referred to an ophthalmologist, who eventually gave her eye crossing a name.

"Strabismus," he said as he handed me another Diagnosis Badge.

Jaycee was barely a year old and I had a collection of badges for diverse diagnoses. I didn't want any more of them, and they were becoming overwhelming. But it didn't matter, the badges kept coming without my ability to stop them.

After some monitoring, it was decided that Jaycee would need surgery on the muscles of her eyes to correct this problem before her brain stopped receiving information from the eye, which was worse. He went on to explain her eye crossing was giving her double-vision, which would affect depth perception, too.

When Jaycee was about 2 years old, she had outpatient surgery on both eyes to correct her strabismus. The surgery was successful, even though we were warned more than one surgery may be warranted. She did have a second surgery for strabismus again when she was 8 years old. Surgery on the eyes sounds uncomfortable, but Jaycee recovered easily from both of them. They were some of the easiest surgeries she ended up having.

After the strabismus diagnosis, we had two years of peace without any new diagnoses. I was hopeful there would be no more given, but it wasn't to be.

Diagnosis Badge Earned: 2009-Obstructive Sleep Apnea

With Jaycee's diagnosis of asthma, a pulmonologist came into our lives to help control her symptoms and frequent respiratory infections. The pulmonologist noticed, as I did, that Jaycee's tonsils were enlarged. They were so big they were "kissing" each other. I often wondered how she ate and drank with those large tonsils!

When Jaycee's heart echocardiograms indicated some slightly high pulmonary pressures, the cardiologist and pulmonologist started to wonder if Jaycee had obstructive sleep apnea, which is common with Down syndrome. At an appointment, I responded to screening questions on a form:

-Does she snore? Not really.
-Is she restless in her sleep? Yes, she flip-flops all over her bed all night.

-Does she stop breathing in her sleep? I don't know. I don't sleep with her.
-Is she tired during the day? Yes, sort of. She's 3-years old and she takes 2-3 hour naps. I'm not sure if that's normal or not.

It was decided Jaycee would need a sleep study to determine if sleep apnea was present. The test itself was worse than I imagined. I was given a short description of the proceedings beforehand and I wondered how feasible it would be on a young child. I figured the hospital must be accustomed to doing the studies on young children like Jaycee, so I wasn't too worried going into the test. I was so unprepared!

Jaycee screamed through the nearly hour-long placement of stickers and probes on various spots on her body, which were glued to her head. She was so frightened and upset; I really hadn't seen her that upset in the hospital. She was completely wired up and she hated it! There were things attached to her head, under her nose, on her chest, on her face, and on her leg—she looked more like a science project than a child. It wasn't like I could rationalize with her, she was only three years old and not yet verbal. She was scared and she wanted it to stop. As her mother, I did, too, even though I knew it was imperative to her health.

Jaycee had a hard time falling asleep for the test, a mandatory aspect for a sleep study. After all, she was not in her own room or comfortable with everything connected to her. She eventually did drift off much later than usual, but she woke up so distressed a few hours into the test and got physically sick. I was surprised by her reaction, and I felt I was doing a poor job of comforting my daughter during the test. The sleep technician was ready to call the study off, however, I convinced her to let us stay and I tried my best to get her calmed down and back to sleep. I was quite frustrated the technician didn't seem to be interested in helping me calm my child down. Perhaps she didn't know what to do, but neither did I! I knew the results were important to determine if she had obstructive sleep apnea or if there was an issue with her heart. When Jaycee finally settled down, she slept long enough for them to get the data they needed. We were both so glad when the sleep study was over!

The results came back just as the pulmonologist and cardiologist believed, obstructive sleep apnea. I was not surprised given the size of Jaycee's tonsils. The next step would be removing those giant tonsils and adenoids, which for most people. fixes the problem. I was sure it would help my daughter, so I didn't take this Diagnosis Badge seriously, since I felt it was only temporary.

After the surgery and difficult recovery time (remember Elijah's birth story), another sleep study was conducted to verify the surgery had "fixed" her obstructive sleep apnea. Once again, I found myself in the sleep lab with Jaycee, but this time I was prepared to make her comfortable with her favorite movies, toys, and her grandma. I had an arsenal of distractions available to help her forget about all the stuff she was hooked up to for the study. Her reaction to the whole process went better than the first, which was my prayer.

A few weeks later, a nurse called to tell me the results indicated that Jaycee still had obstructive sleep apnea. *What?* That wasn't supposed to happen. The diagnosis initially made sense given her huge tonsils, but when they were gone, and the diagnosis remained, it caught me off guard. At the time, Jaycee was not overweight, which is often another contributor. I wasn't really prepared to take the badge permanently, but there it was, one more to add to my sash.

Since the surgery did not "cure" Jaycee's obstructive sleep apnea, a CPAP machine was recommended. When Jaycee started using this machine as a 3-year-old, I expected that, as she aged, she would eventually outgrow the problem. I was wrong yet again. The machine has never left its place in her bedroom, and this Diagnosis Badge never left my sash.

Perhaps, the hope of Jaycee outgrowing certain diagnoses helped me cope with them better. I had to accept some of them slowly over time. If I thought my child would have a CPAP machine from age three to forever, it just seemed too overwhelming. It was much easier to hope that it was temporary. I eventually came to realize she was never going to have a normal sleep study result. It took me years to accept this diagnosis was permanent and I gave up hope for a different outcome.

This diagnosis proved to be more serious than I had initially thought. The sleep apnea, in combination with her heart issue and asthma, made colds dangerous. Her breathing at night was usually compromised first during illnesses because of her apnea. However, another more serious threat was on its way a few years later.

By: Evana Sandusky

Diagnosis Badge Earned: January 2011-Wolff-Parkison-White Syndrome

There are some days that start off innocent and mundane but then turn into completely horrible life-changing moments. On this seemingly normal day in January, my husband was off from work and at home caring for Elijah and Jaycee. Jaycee, who was almost five years old, was home sick from pre-school. We weren't sure what was wrong with her, but she wasn't acting like herself. Neither of us were too worried about Jaycee that morning I left for work. I went to work knowing Jason would call if anything went wrong.

I am a speech-language pathologist who works with children, mostly toddlers, with delays in their homes. I was scheduled for a home therapy session just a few miles from our house. As usual for this particular family, they weren't home for our session. I would later see this as a blessing, but at the time it was an annoyance. I took advantage of the free hour at home since I was so close and had a chance to see Jaycee and grab some lunch. I hate working while she's sick; I'm always nervous something is going to happen when I'm away. So, I was happy to have a moment to look in on Jaycee myself before going back to work that afternoon.

I grilled Jason on Jaycee's status when I arrived home. Is she going to the bathroom? Eating? What did you try to feed her? Drinking? Fever? He wasn't concerned with her symptoms, but he did say she was tired. In fact, she couldn't eat lunch because she was falling asleep at the table. That was very unusual, but I decided to eat a quick salad and let Jaycee rest before I disturbed her by thoroughly checking her over myself.

When I walked in Jaycee's room ten minutes later, I was immediately worried. She was fast asleep—at noon. That was very odd. She was also pale; her skin was usually almost red, for reasons I can't explain, so her paleness was alarming to me. I tried to rouse her awake, but she was so lethargic. I had never seen her like this.

I put her oxygen saturation monitor on her, which we had in our possession thanks to her obstructive sleep apnea. I hoped the monitor would reveal why she looked so bad. She didn't seem to be having difficulty breathing but there had been a few occasions where she wasn't wheezing but couldn't breathe easily. Her oxygen saturation level was normal, but her heart rate was 235.

"That can't be right!"

I knew a "fast" rate for Jaycee was 150-180. I thought the signal was bad or the machine was broken. I tried putting the heart rate monitor on a different finger. I had Jason reattach the sensor and then again, we couldn't make sense of what we were seeing. There was no way her heart rate was that fast! I lifted her shirt to look at her chest. I could literally see her chest pounding and a vein in her neck was pulsating. Could that number be correct? What in the world was going on with her?

I called our local doctor and spoke to the nurse, as I couldn't comprehend the new problem. I guess I should have known to go the emergency room, but things were not processing as fast as they should have. I had planned on popping in for lunch and heading back to work; I wasn't ready for this scene and new set of symptoms. The nurse told us to go to a specific hospital, so we grabbed the kids and loaded them into the car. Elijah was just a year old and we were once again in a new crisis with him in tow. Jaycee was so weak that we had to carry her to the vehicle. She didn't have the strength to sit up either. It was one of the few times we rushed her to the ER without buckling her up in her seat belt. I sat in the back of the truck with Jaycee, watching the monitor the whole way as well as directly at her for other signs of life. Her eyes were open and she made small movements, but it was obvious something was seriously wrong. We planned to go to a bigger hospital about 40 minutes away as advised, but I got scared a few minutes into the drive and pleaded with my husband to go to our local, rural hospital. I was afraid Jaycee wouldn't make it if we decided to go any farther. I had brushed up on CPR when Jaycee was born years ago, but I didn't want to have to use it.

Perhaps you are wondering why we didn't call an ambulance. In our rural community, we can drive to the hospital faster than waiting for the ambulance. I know that may be hard to believe, but it is the truth. I'm pretty sure that's why the nurse didn't tell me to call for an ambulance. I know family members who have waited for 40 minutes or more on an ambulance to arrive at their home.

In that amount of time, they could have been at the hospital getting help. Thanks to my husband's driving, we were at the ER in record time.

Upon arrival, I carried Jaycee in my arms, walking as fast as I could to the ER check-in while Jason parked the truck and carried in little Elijah. In this little emergency room, we had to get buzzed inside through a locked door to tell someone why we were there seeking treatment. I frantically pushed the button trying to call someone to the door. My daughter was having a true emergency after all!

A female nurse opened the door just enough to poke her out to tell me something like, "We are completely full. You're going to have to wait to be seen." No, she was not going to triage my daughter or even ask why we were there. Then she glanced down at Jaycee and said, "What's wrong with her anyway?" She seemed to notice that Jaycee looked lifeless.

"Her heart rate is 235," I said.

"Well, how do you know it's that fast?" the nurse asked. I sensed she didn't believe me. It was an annoying but fair question. I guess most people don't have monitors at home to check that sort of thing. By this time in Jaycee's life, I had made numerous trips to the emergency room; the thing I discovered was most staff members seem to assume you are not having an emergency but are most likely an overreacting parent, until proven otherwise. I was prepared to say anything or burst into tears if necessary to get her seen immediately.

As soon as I gave the nurse more information, we were immediately escorted back to a room, though it wasn't really a designated patient room. On the way to the impromptu waiting area, I glanced into the actual waiting room; the nurse wasn't lying--they were full. In the room, a heart monitor was put on Jaycee, which showed a faster rate than our monitor had. The number 256 flashed on the screen. That number was twenty beats faster and much scarier than the one we measured. The nurse seemed surprised and yelled for the doctor, who was busy with other patients, to quickly come care for my daughter.

In a short time, they shuffled patients and made a room available for Jaycee. Hospital staff soon flooded the room, which frightened me because I didn't know what was happening. I am sure some of the staff were just as concerned as I was, since they knew our family well. They weren't sure what exactly was happening since Jaycee had never had this problem before, though no one offered an explanation to me anyway. I didn't know the severity of the situation right away. Sometimes ignorance helps.

The staff phoned Jaycee's cardiologist and got information on how to proceed. Jason stayed with Elijah in the waiting room until my parents arrived shortly after us. Thankfully, Jason was sitting in the room with us when we learned they were sending a helicopter to transport Jaycee to St. Louis. Actually, we were standing. I don't recall sitting down during this long ordeal until it was over, which ended up being a couple of hours later.

After we found out about the transport, my husband went home with Elijah and my father to pack a hospital bag for us and a suitcase for our son to stay with grandma. While he was gone, the seriousness of the situation became known, and I regretted sending Jason away for something as meaningless as clothes.

While we were waiting for the helicopter, a plan was made to administer a medication to bring her heart rate down. If it didn't work within a few minutes, they would give the medication again. The danger was that the medication could make her heart rate become too slow. A crash cart was wheeled into the room in case it was needed. The staff were doing their best to think ahead of the possible scenarios that may result, since no one knew how Jaycee would react.

When I overheard the staff preparing for different outcomes and saw the crash cart, my heart sank. *This was not good.* No one was really telling me too much about the situation because they were all busy working. It became apparent things were bad.

Jaycee looked at me occasionally with tired eyes. I put my terrified feelings aside. I wanted to hug her and wail. I could not believe my baby was going through another traumatic event at such a young age. There were a dozen people around working, and I needed to be strong for Jaycee and everyone in the room. I held her hand tightly and kissed her hand and her head. I didn't say much because I had a lump in my throat that blocked any words that wanted to come out. When I could muster a word or two, I spoke them to her while looking at the monitors and hoping to see a

By: Evana Sandusky

different number. My mom stood next to the bed praying for Jaycee and telling her everything was going to be fine.

I silently prayed, "God, is this how it's all going to end? This is so unpredictable and unexpected. This can't be how it ends!! Help her!"

Again, I hated myself in that moment for sending Jason away for clothes. Who cares about clean clothes for tomorrow when your daughter may not live in the next few minutes? I called him and told him to get back immediately. He informed me the packing was nearly complete and he had time to finish. I told him to drop everything he was doing and get back now—a crash cart was on stand-by. Then he understood and returned about 10 minutes later, missing all the excitement that would happen next.

The time came for the medication push. My mom and I held Jaycee's hands. My mom continued to pray. I, along with everyone else in the room, stared at the monitors. The medication went in and there was no change in her heart rate. Nothing! My heart sank. It didn't work. The status was relayed to the cardiologist on the phone. I heard them shouting out information back and forth to the person on the phone and the people in the room.

A few minutes later, the medication was pushed again. Her heart rate started to go down and then rapidly it went too low. It was a split second, but it felt longer. There were moans in the room and I believe I yelled, "No!" as if my word could somehow stop her heart rate from going dangerously low. But as quickly as it dropped, it went back up. It was around 180 beats, which was high but no longer extremely dangerous. The medication worked, and everyone sighed with relief. Many of the hospital staff knew us personally since our town is small, and they were glad to see the positive result.

My husband arrived just when all that excitement was over. I sat (finally) in a chair feeling weak and trying to process the last couple of hours. The salad I ate hours earlier churned violently in my stomach. A nurse saw I didn't look well and put a trashcan near me; I never had to use it, thankfully.

About the time the helicopter transport team arrived, one test showed that Jaycee was positive for Influenza A. She had a flu shot previously, but it apparently didn't protect her. Jaycee was loaded up in the helicopter while Jason and I raced to St. Louis in our vehicle. We were warned she might have another episode of her heart racing during the transport but the medics stated they were prepared. I was scared. I wondered if she would still be alive when we got to the hospital. The two-hour drive felt like torture and my mind tried to supply pictures of what I would be walking into when we saw her next. My mind always creates a worse-case scenario than what ends up happening.

At the hospital, we were not able to see her regular cardiologist but did see other ones that were working on the floor. They determined she had a tachycardia brought on by the Influenza A virus. The doctors claimed it was a one-time event and wouldn't happen again—they were confident. We were instructed to follow up with her regular cardiologist within about a week. Jaycee was discharged a few days later without having any more problems. We all went home, shaken by the whole situation but relieved it was just a fluke reaction to the virus.

Soon after, we found ourselves meeting with Jaycee's regular cardiologist. He reviewed the information and performed his own set of tests during his office visit. We knew this man well so when he shut the door, looked sad, and took a seat beside us, I wondered what could be wrong.

Wolff-Parkinson-White (WPW) syndrome was explained to us. Basically, Jaycee had an extra electrical pathway in her heart; when it fired, she would have another event of her heart racing. Since she had one tachycardia, she would most certainly have another one. It might be in two days, two months, or 20 years. No one can predict what would set it off or when it would happen, but it would occur again. WPW is serious because it can cause sudden death.

Sudden death? That didn't sound optimistic. This Diagnosis Badge felt like a heavy burden on my sash.

Jaycee was immediately put on a beta-blocker, as a preventative measure, with the understanding that a tachycardia could occur even on this medication. A heart ablation was scheduled a few months later. The ablation was the best and only way to fix her heart to prevent this from happening again. An ablation entails inserting a catheter (tube) into a vein through the groin up to the heart; the area that is causing the problem is then destroyed by a radiofrequency to stop the rapid heart rate. Jason and I understood that sometimes more than one ablation was needed to effectively treat WPW.

I counted down the days to the ablation. Each day Jaycee lived with WPW was mentally exhausting for me. Knowing there was a possibility of the tachycardia happening before the procedure occurred was small but still, it was there along with the possibility of death. It was the most mentally straining time as we were living with the fear our child might die at any moment. It was really months of mental torture for me.

I was filled with happiness on the day of the ablation. Usually procedures and surgeries made me nervous but, in this case, I was ready to put this behind us. I was ready to have normal days with Jaycee again, when I didn't have to worry about her suddenly dying.

Initially, the procedure was considered a success. I gladly removed that weighty Diagnosis Badge. But the one-month post ablation testing indicated the pathway had healed itself and was back. Yet another blow! In an instant, the burden of the badge was back on. The fears, the questions, the stress, the uncertainty that came with the badge took root in me again. Some people do need a second ablation, but we were hoping Jaycee wouldn't be one of these. We were told the WPW was back, but they had no way of determining if it would be capable of causing her heart to race again. It might never cause a tachycardia again but then again, it might. It was a gamble that our cardiologist didn't think we should take given the fact Jaycee had one episode in her life already.

A few months later, the ablation was repeated and was successful. The WPW Diagnosis Badge was off my sash once again and for good.

Though the badge is no longer visible and active, there is an imprint on my sash from the badge that will forever remain. The memory of those events is still powerful and reminds me that Jaycee's life is so precious.

Diagnosis Badge Earned: Spring 2014-Severe GERD

We endured a few years without a new Diagnosis Badge. However, Jaycee was not in good health during that time. She had struggled with illness after illness, and I was beyond frustrated with her health and the lack of concern from her specialists.

I decided a second opinion was necessary to see if there was anything that had been overlooked with Jaycee. I sat in a hospital three and a half hours away from home with Jaycee, now 8-years old, to receive my next badge. Jaycee had just undergone a rigorous evaluation from a Complex Aero-Digestive Evaluation Team whose goal was to find possible reasons for her frequent and recurrent pneumonia. An ear-nose-throat doctor, gastroenterologist, and a pulmonary doctor scoped, tested, and biopsied Jaycee from her mouth to her intestines. Fortunately, Jaycee was under anesthesia for the numerous tests, so she handled it all like a pro. If there was something to find, I was confident it would be.

The major new diagnosis after all that testing was GERD (gastroesophageal reflux disease). Before the pH impendence probe confirmed the reflux, I was completely unaware she was having any trouble in this area. The screening questions beforehand did not raise any concerns with me either. She did not have frequent spitting up, coughing with or after meals, frequent burping, or changes in vocal quality after eating; however, Jaycee was minimally verbal, so she didn't use her voice enough for me to notice any changes, if there were any. She could not communicate pain, heartburn, or any similar internal symptom due to her limited speech. The doctor said there was a very small percentage of children with silent reflux who have no outward signs and wanted to rule this out for Jaycee. Neither he nor I had concerns going into the reflux testing.

When the impendence probe indicated that Jaycee had reflux during the day and nearly all night long, I was alarmed. How could I not know? I wondered how long Jaycee had been silently dealing with this problem. Was she in pain often? Then I thought about all of Jaycee's favorite foods, which we frequently ate like spaghetti, pizza, tacos, and salsa. They were all triggers for reflux, which may have, unbeknownst to me, been causing her more reflux problems. This girl loves to eat salsa with a spoon! I couldn't believe it!

By: Evana Sandusky

The evaluation team did not feel the reflux was causing Jaycee's frequent pneumonia, but it certainly wasn't good for her body given the large amount of inflammation present. They estimated she had been having reflux for quite a while when looking at her tissue.

The first step after this diagnosis was adding an oral medication. I was confident this medication could treat her reflux, and all would be fine. After Jaycee had been on the medication for a few months, she was brought back to the hospital for a second pH impendence probe to verify the medication was treating her reflux.

The first time the probe was place down her nose and into her esophagus, she was sedated while other tests were performed. This time, she would be awake, and we would be in the room with her while it was inserted.

I was truly unprepared for this procedure, much like that first nightmare sleep study Jaycee went through years earlier. Before the probe was placed, Jaycee, my mother, and I talked with the nurse practitioner (NP) who apparently did these probe placements all the time. We warned her that Jaycee would fight the probe and asked for people to be ready to hold her down, though. We didn't necessarily want to be one of those people. The NP assured me that everyone would be ready for Jaycee and not to worry, as the placement wouldn't take very long.

We were led back to a sterile room and waited for the radiologist to arrive, who would take an x-ray to confirm the probe was placed correctly in the esophagus. There was no one else in the room, against our best advice. She did not recruit anyone to help us hold Jaycee down, even though she assured us she would. I figured more people would come in after the radiologist was ready, but I was wrong.

The radiologist arrived and took his position. My mom and I suddenly found ourselves holding down a screaming and crying Jaycee on a flat table as the NP started running the probe down her nose. Before we knew it, it was starting. Jaycee was gagging and coughing as this "professional" lady jabbed this probe in her nose and tried to run it down the back of her mouth. To me, the NP looked like she was being rough. Jaycee's nose was bleeding, she wet herself, and she was fighting as hard as she could. The NP kept telling Jaycee to swallow so the probe would go down. My mom and I both kept saying back to her that she didn't understand and was too upset to follow directions. Finally, the probe went where it was supposed to go, and my mom and I wondered what just happened. There was no preparation for any of us and no regard was given to Jaycee's emotions or her other developmental factors.

I was irate; I couldn't talk. I should have told the NP that making family members hold down their child and witness that placement was inappropriate. I should have yelled at her for promising to have people help hold Jaycee down when she obviously had no intentions to get such people. I couldn't though because I was too busy trying to calm and console Jaycee and trying to clean up the blood and urine on her. Vomit was added to the list of bodily fluids on Jaycee before we left the hospital—and that was my breaking point.

By that time in my life, I had seen Jaycee poked, prodded, tested, and hooked up to many, many different things. That pH probe placement was by far the most horrific outpatient procedure we have ever experienced. I hated myself for putting Jaycee through that and for not telling that NP how unprofessional the whole situation was, but especially her demeanor and actions. I never wanted to be a part of holding her down for the placement. I wanted to be the person holding her hand trying to keep her calm, not the monster forcing her to undergo emotional and physical pain. My mom, Jaycee, and I all felt traumatized as we left the hospital.

The worst part of that whole process came afterwards. While wearing the probe for 24 hours, Jaycee came down with pneumonia, which was confirmed by an x-ray. The results of the pH probe eventually indicated that her reflux was worse after starting the medication, but the doctors decided to throw out the study due to her pneumonia and subsequent vomiting that occurred during the study. The solution to this "bad study" was... yep, another pH impedance probe study! I consented but I was adamant about Jaycee being given a sedative to help calm her and for Jaycee to be treated under better conditions. I then vented all my pent-up frustrations as I complained about the NP and our previous experience to the scheduler on the phone. I *would not* let Jaycee be treated so poorly again. The third (and last) pH impedance placement went much better, and we were all thankful for that. The third study revealed Jaycee's reflux had not improved. . In fact, there really wasn't much of a difference now that she was taking medication. She was still having reflux day and night. Her longest reflux lasted an hour and a half while she was sleeping! Several options were discussed, but ultimately, we decided to continue with the medications and adjust her lifestyle.

GERD started off seeming like not a big deal compared to other medical issues in Jaycee's life. But then again, it's hard to know how much it bothered Jaycee given that she couldn't communicate her problems and pain.

To fight GERD, we elevated her bed, so her head would be a little higher. I started making meals that were safer for her. I whipped up chicken spaghetti or Alfredo instead of regular tomato-based spaghetti. Tacos and salsa became a rare food instead of a weekly one. Chocolate, in any form, was given to her as a special, rare treat and not chosen if there was an alternative; however, most of the chocolate candy Jaycee received for holidays had to be confiscated. Later, these lifestyle changes, along with increasing her dose of medications, did show improvement in her reflux, which made all the modifications worthwhile. This diagnosis brought about some unexpected traumatic testing, dietary changes, and a new specialist in our lives.

My sash was filling up with Diagnoses Badges, each with a significant day attached to it. I'll never forget the days associated when my daughter received her diagnoses nor the emotions I endured for her. Both of our lives changed on those days although my emotions regarding them changed over time. Still, other badges would be coming too.

By: Evana Sandusky

CHAPTER 3:

THE HOSPITAL CARE BADGE

> *Hospital Care Badge: When a child is admitted to the hospital for a surgery or an illness, the mother earns this badge while caring for her child in the hospital. Only one badge is earned per child, even though the mother might care for her child on more than one occasion. This badge is only given for hospital admissions that do not include unplanned time in the intensive care unit.*

Hospital Care Badge Earned: 2006

After Jaycee was born, we knew she would be admitted to the hospital for her first open heart surgery as an infant. Jaycee's congestive heart failure and pulmonary hypertension was being treated with medication until surgery. Meanwhile, my job was to get Jaycee's weight from 6 pounds to 9 pounds so that she could have her surgery to correct her AV canal defect. The round-the-clock feedings were not enough for her to gain weight in the desired timeframe. The next step was to change her to a higher calorie formula, since her intake at each feeding was still small, despite my best efforts. That did the trick and soon, she was at the right weight to have the surgery.

There are many things that go through your mind when your baby is about to have major surgery. Getting professional pictures made before surgery was a big priority for me. Just in case something happened to our tiny baby during surgery, I wanted her face and beauty documented. I also wanted pictures of her chest before it became scared forever. As we viewed Jaycee's pictures with the photographer days before surgery, I felt like crying as each photo was shown. Every single pose represented Jaycee "before" so many things, and the future was still unknown.

Another oddity for the hospital stay was packing. I had packed for vacations, church camps, and other fun activities, but I had never packed for something like this before. I wasn't sure what to pack, especially which baby supplies I would need to bring along. How many outfits were required to bring in case her stay was longer than expected? It was a surreal moment that caused stress and reminded me that my motherhood role was more diverse than most.

The stress leading up to the surgery was nothing like I had ever experienced. Her care was intense and exhausting. I was also dealing with post-pregnancy hormones and adjusting to Jaycee's life-long diagnosis of Down syndrome. There was so much to be concerned about, I didn't know where to start. I was so worried about her life and future.

Still, I prayed. Our church prayed. We had everyone and anyone pray for Jaycee to make it through the obstacles in her short life. Honestly, we prayed for a miracle, for her heart to be supernaturally healed. But the echocardiogram the day before the surgery showed the large hole was still there. I am not sure why the technician said, "Well, the AV canal defect is still there. She will need the surgery tomorrow. I know that's not what you want to hear." We never told him we were hoping for a miracle. Perhaps, every parent comes in hoping for a supernatural healing, so the tech provides that speech to all parents. I'm not sure why, but for whatever reason, that man's words gave me peace.

The next day was surgery day, and I was as prepared as I could be. Jaycee was such a happy, three-month-old baby; she had no idea what was in store for her that morning. Jason and I spent time cuddling her, giving her kisses, and trying not to think about what was going to happen to her little body in a few minutes. Before we knew it, the time to hand her off and let the hospital staff take over came. Even though I cried after her departure, I was at peace. I was both dreading this moment and wanting to get it over with at the same time.

Jaycee's grandparents and other members of our support team were in the waiting area. We prayed and took communion with our pastor during the wait. The surgery lasted four hours, which felt like the longest ones of my life at that point. When the doctor emerged from the surgery and deemed it a success, we were all relieved.

Seeing Jaycee after the surgery was shocking. She was hooked up to even more machines than when she was in the NICU. Her chest tube was probably the worst thing to see after surgery, as it made Jaycee look so fragile. I was glad she made it through the surgery but was also worried about her recovery. This was all so new and at times overwhelming.

Jaycee spent six nights in the hospital before being discharged to go home. I spent my days in the hospital feeding Jaycee bottles and holding her. The rest of the time was spent waiting for wires and tubes to be removed from her body as she healed. My husband and I talked to her and made sure her favorite toys from home were always within reach. If she fell asleep, we snuck out of the room for a break and to eat. If she was awake, we made sure Jaycee could see us, so she would know she was not alone.

Jaycee's recovery seemed to go as planned, except for one thing. Jaycee was eating as well as she was before the surgery and she looked alert and awake, but she needed a whiff of oxygen, 0.1 liters to be exact. When she couldn't be weaned off, it was decided she would go home on oxygen, which she ended up needing for the next three months.

When I earned that Hospital Care Badge, I foolishly thought it would be one of the last times we'd ever be in the hospital with Jaycee. I had no idea just how many opportunities I would have to keep this badge fresh.

Another Stitch for the Hospital Care Badge

Being in the hospital for a planned surgery is one thing but being in the hospital for an unexpected illness is something different all together. When Jaycee had her heart surgery, we had a specific date and were able to arrange for our household to be in order and to pack a suitcase that was well thought out. When Jaycee suddenly became sick, the hospital became a new experience for us. An emergency illness is dissimilar to a preplanned one as everything is done chaotically.

At a year old, Jaycee had caught a simple cold and was wheezing. Days passed, and she just wasn't getting any better. We saw her pediatrician once or twice in the office before finally deciding to go to the emergency room. Not choosing to go to the hospital just six miles from our house, since it's mainly for adult patients, we drove to the next closest hospital, about 35 miles away, knowing they cared for some children as well as adults.

We arrived in the emergency room and were taken back quickly. The nurse remarked at how much Jaycee was wheezing. Her oxygen saturation monitor showed a number in the upper 80s. I stupidly asked the nurse, "Are you going to admit her?" I don't have to ask that question for the most part now because I know the cut off for certain vital signs that necessitate an admission. At the time though, I had so much to learn about illnesses and how the health care system worked. Of course, Jaycee was admitted and given a diagnosis of pneumonia. It was our first taste of caring for a child in the hospital unexpectantly. My husband and I both took off from work and stayed with her almost constantly, since this illness really scared us. I slept in the room with her, reassured her, and kept track of her meals and medications. Even back then, I felt I needed to make sure people were giving her good care as I didn't trust other people to manage her care and respond to her like I would. They weren't me, and she needed me—her mother. It seemed weird to leave her, too. I always had a problem with that.

We didn't know how Jaycee should have been monitored or what the treatment should have been since this was new territory for us. We were ignorant and at the mercy of those trying to take

By: Evana Sandusky

care of her. Looking back, the people in that hospital did the best they could, but they were not a children's hospital. They didn't have the information, training, or equipment needed for Jaycee's recovery. Nor were they prepared to deal with a child with Down syndrome, a repaired heart defect, and asthma. So, I will just say that mistakes were made which we alerted them to, such as forgetting to turn her oxygen back on after a nebulizer treatment. After several days of treating Jaycee unsuccessfully, they agreed she needed to be transferred to a children's hospital for specialized care. That led to Jaycee having her first ambulance ride. Her baby book filled up with bizarre firsts like that.

The care she got at the St. Louis Children's Hospital was outrageous. She went from an oxygen tent to oxygen through a nasal cannula. Plus, her oxygen levels were monitored 24/7 instead of just random spot checks. We asked questions, tried to make sense of this illness, and hoped it wouldn't happen again. There is a learning curve to being in the hospital, and we were eager to learn everything we could to help Jaycee.

Keep on Stitching for the Badge

The learning continued with more and more unplanned hospital admissions since that first time. Jaycee was a patient in the hospital numerous times for a variety of reasons. Occasionally, Jaycee was admitted for something simple going completely wrong. There was a short admission after a complication from a diagnostic heart catheterization, and a blood clot and respiratory distress showed me that a routine procedure has very real risks.

Most of Jaycee's hospital admissions have been for respiratory issues like asthma, pneumonia, and viruses. Some of the hospital stays were for four or five days while others were over a week or more. Most of the time, Jaycee needs to be in the hospital because her oxygen saturation levels have gotten low at home, which means she needs oxygen temporarily and frequent breathing treatments.

Caring for Jaycee in the hospital is even more stressful. Over time, I have learned the difference between when Jaycee is sick and not recovering as expected versus when she's sick but making progress in the hospital. In other words, I have been well-educated in when I need to be extremely worried about her condition and when I can care for her from home. Obviously, if she's in the hospital, her body is struggling to fight off something on its own, so things are not going super great. But it is different if she just needs an increase in medications and a little bit of oxygen for a few days to get her over the hump versus being on ventilation support and not being allowed to eat because she's too sick. That kind of knowledge of how to gage when things are bad comes only with multiple admissions. There's always an underlying concern about Jaycee's health whenever she's in the hospital. It may be a large or a small concern, but it's there, as no matter what is happening, she is my daughter first and foremost.

When Jaycee is in the hospital, I handle some of her care, which comes with the badge and motherhood. I help with her bathing, dressing, and eating, just like a normal day at home. It helps me feel like I'm still doing something productive as her mother even though nurses are there to assist if she's hooked up to several machines or lines. The older Jaycee gets, the more she prefers that I do these personal tasks for her. She doesn't appreciate a stranger diapering her when she is confined to a hospital bed but tolerates me better. I also hold Jaycee when she's upset and talk to her when she's crying, just as any mother would, except in our case there are not many "just as" days.

There are times though when she's really upset during a not-so-pleasant procedure and I just have to walk away. Some things required for her health care I don't want to see or remember. I must safeguard myself, too, and let the professionals do their jobs. I once witnessed a PICC line (a catheter going from the arm to the heart for long-term IV medication, nutrition, and blood drawing) being taken out of her arm and decided I didn't need to see that again.

Keeping Jaycee well-stocked in movies was another job of mine. I raided the hospital movie cabinets to find her favorite characters in movies and searched Netflix for shows she might enjoy. Yes, these jobs are important for Jaycee, and for me, during a hospital stay. I need to feel like I'm still her mom, and she needs to know I'm there for her.

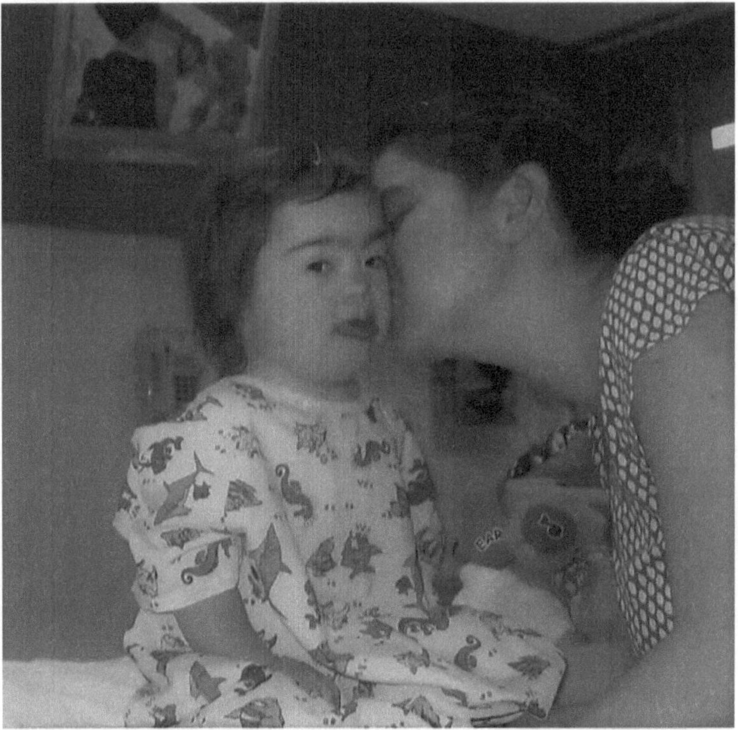

Getting a Kiss from Mommy Before Surgery in 2008

When we are in the St. Louis Children's Hospital, which is located a solid two hours from our home, life continues. Caring for Jaycee in the hospital doesn't mean the jobs at home stop. When an admission happens, I must tie up things with my job by canceling appointments and making sure nothing pressing needs to be done. I must make sure the mail is collected and the bills are paid. Beyond that, I have to have clean clothes to wear in the hospital. Fortunately, the hospital we use has a couple of places to do laundry for free. In short, a mom is still busy being a mom, even in the hospital.

When Elijah was born, I had a new concern. How would I care for one child in the hospital and meet the needs of one child at home? When I had Elijah, I realized I would probably have to leave him to care for Jaycee in the hospital. I hoped that day would be far off in the future. That was not to be. When Elijah was just five months old, Jaycee was admitted to the hospital for pneumonia. It was hard leaving Elijah, but fortunately it was only for a few days. I'm thankful Elijah and Jaycee's grandparents all live close to us, as well as her aunt and uncle, who can help with Elijah's care on short notice.

Almost every time I leave Elijah to bring Jaycee to the hospital, I feel torn. I hope he won't hold it against me later in life, but Jaycee takes a priority when she's in the hospital. I have always tried to explain things to Elijah in words he can understand so he has some idea of why mom isn't around. As he has gotten older, we've been able to stay in touch through phone calls or video chats. Depending on Jaycee's illness, Elijah will visit us in the hospital for a few hours or sometimes a few days, staying with one of us at a hotel. When he does come, I am often drained by his energy. I try my hardest to still be a mother to both children while one is in the hospital. It is a juggling act and one I have been forced to attempt.

By: Evana Sandusky

The Hospital Care Badge represents the child's illness that both mom and child survived. It is a heavy badge full of emotions, vivid memories, decisions, separations, and perseverance. Though it was one I hoped to return very early on, it still has its place on my sash, and probably always will.

CHAPTER 4:

THE ICU BADGE

> *Intensive Care Unit Badge: When a child is admitted into the intensive care unit due to an unexpectant illness, injury, or accident, the mother earns this badge while caring for her child in the hospital's ICU. Due to the seriousness of an ICU stay, a new badge is earned every time the child is admitted into the ICU.*

ICU Badge Earned: February 2006

Jaycee's birth introduced us to the world of the neonatal intensive care unit (NICU). Jaycee was initially transferred to a hospital with a NICU the night she was born by a helicopter (That transport would later introduce us to the scary world of medical bills.). The NICU is where we found out about Jaycee's Down syndrome and AV canal defect. It was also where we were introduced to monitors, hospital jargon, and common hospital practices.

The NICU was an unexpected world we landed in with Jaycee. It was where we observed the first of many IV placements and painful blood draws. It was the first of many experiences we had waiting to hear test results. It was also the first time we saw Jaycee on oxygen and our daughter receive medications. These firsts are not expected by parents when you are preparing to have a baby.

In the NICU, Jaycee was treated for several health issues. She needed oxygen because her oxygen saturation levels were low without it. She did not take to breastfeeding well initially; for Jaycee's sake, they were discontinued, as she physically couldn't do it and every calorie counted. Within a few days, bottle feedings were somewhat successful. Jaycee had so much going on and her endurance for feedings was poor, so I was fine letting that motherly desire pass as long as Jaycee was receiving the proper nutrition. Beyond that, Jaycee had jaundice and needed light treatment for five days. It was almost impossible to visit her for more than a few minutes when she was under the bright bilirubin lights, since they were so bright. The first few days of Jaycee's life, which every new mom expects to have at home cuddling her newborn, were spent in a medically-secure environment to ensure her life lasted more than just a few days.

As a mom, the NICU was an odd place to be in with your baby. It felt very unnatural. It was not private since Jaycee was always in a unit with several beds around her. Being in the NICU, there was always one or more nurses around constantly. Instead of bonding privately with Jaycee, we were surrounded by nurses, doctors, other babies, and other parents just like us. When we visited Jaycee in the NICU, we were given one or two uncomfortable chairs to sit in by Jaycee's bed with a full view of the other babies and families around us. I just wanted to be alone with my daughter. I wanted to take all of her in and hold her without getting tangled in wires. I also wasn't confident of my mothering skills, since this was all new to me. First-time mothers are usually apprehensive, but I felt panic-stricken doing anything for the first time with Jaycee since I had so many onlookers. The NICU is a nursery controlled by the medical establishment. Scrubbing in for several minutes just so I could see my baby was reasonable but atypical. The entire NICU was understandably sterile. Without thinking, I once placed my Boppy pillow on the floor for a few seconds while I adjusted my seating position. A nurse saw my mistake and told me anything that touched the floor was officially contaminated and couldn't touch Jaycee. The five-second rule wasn't true in the NICU. There were just so many rules and it made everything I did more intense.

By: Evana Sandusky

I felt like a failure as I carried that unclean Boppy pillow out of the NICU. It was a little thing that blossomed into a big thing, given my hormonal state. Yes, I cried about it. I felt I couldn't do anything right. The breastfeeding was a disaster as well as my attempts at pumping and then I tainted a pillow! Sometimes stressful situations cause unreasonable responses; I definitely had one after the pillow incident.

In addition to all of the other rules, NICU policy dictated when I could and could not see my own baby. There were times the NICU was closed and no one was allowed inside due to procedures or shift changes. All of this made it very difficult for me to bond with Jaycee in those first few precious days. I felt like she wasn't really mine. To combat the range of emotions and stress I was having, I tried to put hats, bibs, and sleepers on that I purchased for Jaycee to make me feel like I was doing something motherly. I wanted to have some say in her life, even if it was just a decision about what hat she wore, it was my decision.

There was so much I didn't get to do with Jaycee in those first few days. It was odd watching nurses give my baby her first bath or feeding her. Diaper changes were often done by the nurses, too, due to all the wires and monitors on Jaycee that made me nervous. These are the little "firsts" that a mom gets to do, but I wasn't the one doing them. Over her 10-day stay, I gradually took part in more of her care under a watchful eye of a nearby nurse. When I was pregnant, I was anxious to handle any newborn since this was my first baby, but Jaycee seemed even more fragile. In the end, I decided it didn't matter who did what as long as Jaycee was getting the care she needed.

It is amazing the discoveries you can make by being outside of your element. The NICU was the place I learned not every nurse is created equal. There were plenty for us to become acquainted with since we usually stayed with Jaycee for hours at a time. Some nurses were gifted teachers and showed compassion for our situation; other nurses made me feel inadequate about caring for my own child. There was one experience in particular in the NICU that was more than upsetting for me.

On one of the first few days of my daughter's life, I was asked to administer an oral medication to Jaycee for the first time. I had never given a baby medication before nor had I ever drawn up a tiny amount. I had no idea what I was doing, but I thought it sounded easy. The nurse observed as Jason and I both practiced drawing up medication dosages before she instructed me to give Jaycee the proper dosage of medication. Actually, there was not precise instructions; I didn't know there was a right way and a wrong way to do it. On the other hand, the nurse clearly knew yet she didn't inform me. I was doomed to fail as soon as I put my thumb on the end of the syringe. I accidently shot all the medication into Jaycee's mouth quickly; Jaycee coughed, gagged, and spit some of the heart medication out. The frustrated nurse responded with something like, "Well, you weren't supposed to use your thumb because you can't control the speed of the administration." Even though it was her poor teaching that caused the error, she made me feel like a failure yet again. I left the NICU and cried wondering how I would care for Jaycee at home. It was an emotional time for me, and nothing seemed to be going right on my end. Jaycee didn't get all her medication that time, but I eventually got it right after some actual instructions from a good nurse. Eventually, I became a pro at giving medication to Jaycee, but then again, I had several opportunities to become better.

After 10 days, Jaycee was deemed well enough to go home. She was drinking enough by mouth and breathing on her own. We had a full schedule of round-the-clock feedings and frequent medication dosages to do once home, but we were glad to finally be in our own familiar surroundings with our new baby.

The ICU Badge was pressed upon my sash next to the other badges I was not expecting to earn so quickly as a mother. I was hopeful this would be my one and only ICU Badge, as it was no place I ever wanted to be again.

ICU Badge Earned: September 2011

When Jaycee left the NICU, we weren't strangers to the hospital. She was back in the ICU a few times for planned recoveries from procedures or surgeries. These admissions were tough, but they were necessary to treat her medical conditions. Planned time in the ICU is different from what I was about to experience over the next few years. When the ICU was planned, I had time to mentally prepare for what Jaycee would endure, what I would see, and how things might progress for all of us. I like plans and schedules and order in my life. Being in the ICU for illnesses allows none of those things. When Jaycee was 5-years old, we had our first unexpected admission to the ICU. It would be a whole new experience for all of us. After a long day at the children's hospital for Jaycee's annual eye examination, we were ready to head home. Jaycee, a pre-school student at the time, hated the examinations at the eye center. The whole day was exhausting because Jaycee fought every bit of it. On top of the rough exam, Jaycee was sick with a cold, though she seemed fine when the day started. On the way home from the hospital, we made some stops to take care of errands. It was a hot, humid day, which is just what Jaycee can't handle. That day, it seemed to bother her even more than usual. We were almost home from our two-hour trip when Jaycee's breathing suddenly seemed labored while riding in the vehicle. She was running a high fever, too. Then she started vomiting, which was a sign for her that things were going downhill quickly.

I talked Jason into stopping in at a local emergency room on the way home. My plan was to get her checked out and get some oral steroids for this asthma flare-up to be set for the weekend. I figured we'd go into the ER, get the script for the medicine, and go home. That was the plan anyway.

This ER experience was just one mess up after another. An X-ray was taken shortly after we saw a doctor but then nothing happened. If you have been to an emergency room, you can relate. We were there for quite a while, watching Jaycee's oxygen saturations decreasing to 88 and her heart rate increasing to 180. I didn't imagine her vital signs would be that poor while we were in the vehicle moments before coming to the ER. These were indications to me that she needed help immediately. She felt hot, but the nurse swore she didn't have a fever, based on the temperature reading from the ear canal thermometer. Unbeknownst to the nurse, those devices have never been accurate for Jaycee, possibly due to her small ear canals. It was obvious to us that Jaycee needed to be on oxygen and have a breathing treatment, both of which were not done. I was hoping she could get some Tylenol for her fever, but my thermometer result didn't matter apparently.

Instead, we just sat there. My husband was getting furious, as was I. The doctor was nowhere to be found and nothing was being done for my daughter. It's very hard to sit in an ER with legitimate concerns and knowledge about your child when no one pays attention. Finally, the nurse appeared with discharge papers telling us she didn't have appendicitis, so we were free to go home. What??!! Appendicitis?

I said, "If we were at the St. Louis Children's Hospital, she'd be on oxygen right now, not being discharged! And we aren't worried about appendicitis, we are worried about her lungs!!"

The nurse backed out of the room and told us he would have someone clarify what was going on. In a short time, a different emergency room doctor was starting his shift. He talked with us, looked at Jaycee's numbers on the monitor, and seemed confused by what he was told by the previous doctor versus what he was looking at. It didn't take much convincing before he was on the phone to the children's hospital.

In a short time, he was back to inform us that the helicopter would be coming to transfer Jaycee to the very place we just left earlier that day. We sort of begged him not to send a helicopter. The bill for a helicopter transport would be extremely high and our insurance coverage for that particular necessity was poor. The thought of the helicopter bill threw us into more of a frenzy. It took years to pay off her rather large helicopter transport bill from the day she was born; we didn't want another bill for thousands of dollars hanging over our heads. We had to wonder, too, if someone would have been giving Jaycee care as soon as we arrived, then maybe a helicopter would not have been needed. So much for my plan and saving money on a transport. We weren't going home with medicine but instead, Jaycee was sick enough to be admitted and we were going to have financial stress on top of it. The call to transport her by helicopter was up to the doctors at the children's hospital to make and couldn't be undone. It was happening despite our pleas.

Imagine being told you are going home and then a short time later you are told your child is so sick a helicopter transport is needed. It was very surreal. These are some of the reasons why I question doctors and speak up if I'm worried. Doctors are human beings, and humans make mistakes. I'm just glad the second doctor took time to listen to us and examine Jaycee again. The transport team arrived a short time later. Even though we hated the idea of a transport, we were so glad to see people who understood that Jaycee needed oxygen and basic care and took steps to

By: Evana Sandusky

help her finally. Their thermometer showed she had a high fever and they ordered Tylenol immediately. I wasn't crazy, the other thermometer wasn't working properly. The transport team seemed just as infuriated as Jason and me. They started ordering medications and getting things started before the flight even took off. Jaycee was admitted straight to the ICU. We were accustomed to her being in the hospital but not the ICU. It was scary for us to realize Jaycee was sick enough for the ICU when she seemed fine after her eye exam. We began to wonder if she was going to die. Being in the ICU for an illness was new territory for us. It brought out many fears. We didn't understand the levels of need in the ICU, so just being there was terrifying. Jaycee had pneumonia in both lungs and needed a large amount of oxygen. She eventually got up to 11 liters of oxygen, which seemed like a lot to me (It is by the way.). With her oxygen requirement being so high, she was switched to full-time BiPAP support, a machine similar to her CPAP machine at home. I had never heard of a child needing to wear a BiPAP while awake because he or she was having trouble breathing. I didn't understand what was happening and it worried me.

I made the mistake of asking what support came next if the BiPAP support didn't work. The nurse informed me that intubation would be next, which caused me to panic. Being ignorant is sometimes good but in this case, it just made me frightened and stressed. I didn't understand how an illness could get this bad in such a small child and short amount of time. Jaycee spent three days on the BiPAP machine, which was only taken off every few hours for a small sip of water. The doctors wouldn't allow her to drink or eat since she was at risk for aspiration.

It was hard to watch her during this time, especially seeing her feel miserable. Jaycee watched television and cried intermittently. I'm sure she was confused and felt horrible. Since she was two-years old, I had been teaching her sign language, and it helped give me some insight into what she was thinking. She signed "drink" often. Then she signed, "Juice, water, milk." She was upset when I denied her requests, as was I. Jaycee also pointed to the IV in her foot and signed "Hurt." This was the first time she communicated pain ever. It was nice to know what she was thinking, so I could try to help her understand what was happening. I signed back to her, "Your lungs are sick. You need a doctor and medicine." Jaycee seemed upset by my words. She didn't understand the gravity of my simple explanation, but she knew she wasn't going home. Once Jaycee got off the breathing machine, she made a quick recovery and was moved out of ICU. I was so thankful she didn't need to be intubated. She spent a total of a week in the hospital to recover. When she was discharged, I was glad to have her back home. I left shaken by the idea that a simple illness could result in Jaycee being in the ICU.

Another ICU Badge Earned: October 2011

A few weeks later, I was still recovering from the emotions I had from the ICU experience. Anxiety and stress I had not experienced since Jaycee's heart surgeries invaded me. I had thought the worst health issues Jaycee faced were over, so I was struggling to deal with the recent set of circumstances. The last hospital admission left me with the fear about her future that I had never considered before this happened.

Before I healed emotionally, Jaycee started to get sick again. It commenced with her usual wheezing and cold symptoms, which now had me on new levels of alertness. I put her asthma action plan medications in effect and prayed. One night she developed a fever, yet her fingers, toes, and lips started to turn blue. We tried giving her the rescue inhaler but saw no improvement. We drove her to the closest emergency room only minutes away (not the one we were just at one month ago that provided inferior care), since her color indicated a severe problem to us. I was really worried about her, especially since she had not been out of the hospital for long. She was given the best treatment in the ER that the hospital could give since it's primarily for adults. Of course, Jaycee needed to go to the children's hospital. This time, and for the first time, a local ambulance oversaw Jaycee's transport. I loaded into the back of the ambulance with Jaycee. I was so worried Jaycee was going to go into the ICU again I was feeling increasingly nauseous. I was just glad this transport was going faster and easier than the last one, but it was not without its problems. The drive over in the ambulance provided more anxiety to an already vexing situation. Instead of giving her oxygen by nasal cannula on the way, she was given blow-by oxygen. Basically, they were just blowing oxygen near her face. I later found out it was due to their lack of a child's-size cannula

They also only spot-checked her oxygen saturation levels, which also concerned me. By that time, I knew Jaycee's numbers could change quickly, so spot checking wouldn't catch an immediate change. Inside I was panicking. I mentioned I was concerned about her breathing to the EMT who quickly reassured me Jaycee was fine. He did another check just to prove that she was and the number was fine, but I wasn't sure if this machine was meant to be used on a five-year-old. Sometimes machines don't give accurate numbers if they aren't used or fitted properly. Again, I was becoming more distrustful of people meant to provide care for Jaycee considering they did not seem prepared or trained enough for a child with a situation as hers. I was relieved when we got to the emergency room at the children's hospital. Jaycee was immediately put on oxygen since her oxygen saturation levels were in the 80s. Perhaps she wasn't fine in the ambulance after all? She needed 8 liters of oxygen! So much for the blow-by oxygen doing any good. One of the ER doctors questioned me on Jaycee's medications. She wanted to know if I was using them properly and how I was administering them. Then she remarked, "Obviously, you need to be trained more on her asthma if she's coming in needing 8 liters of oxygen." I was hurt by those words. I felt like a horrible mother—once more.

I began second-guessing myself and everything I had done in the past few days. This doctor put the blame on me, and I didn't need any extra blame. I wish she would have yelled at the people who transported us over. It could have been that Jaycee's condition worsened in the past few hours we spent at the unequipped adult hospital and ambulance. Jaycee didn't receive the appropriate care she needed for the past few hours, but this doctor felt it was due to my inexperience. ERs were proving to be terrible places; either I was seen like an overreacting parent or an incompetent mother withholding medical treatment. I couldn't believe it! Needless to say, Jaycee went straight up to ICU for the second time in two months. We learned Jaycee had pneumonia in one lung. She went on the BiPAP full-time again for a couple of days. It was very similar to the month before. Quite frankly, this admission alarmed me. What was happening to Jaycee that made her end up in the ICU two months in a row? Why was she so symptomatic to pneumonia? Was there something else wrong with her that wasn't discovered yet? Did she need to be taken out of school? Is she going to end up back here soon? I had a thousand questions and no answers.

I wasn't the only one thinking some of these questions either. The doctors were also concerned that she was back in again. She was tested for cystic fibrosis—negative. We met with immunology who ran a few tests that yielded nothing alarming. There didn't seem to be a good explanation for the illnesses except that she just kept catching things that were difficult for her body to fight off, given her health history. That explanation was not good enough for me. If there was no explanation, then there was nothing I could do to prevent it from happening again. Everything was out of our control. Still, the doctors encouraged me that it was safe for Jaycee to continue in school.

Jaycee spent about five days in intensive care on the BiPAP and then was weaned down on her oxygen support. Then she was transferred to the floor for a few days before coming home. Jaycee didn't go back to school immediately as I tried to give her body time to recover, fearing she would catch something else. I never expected to be getting an ICU Badge again so soon, but there it was on my sash. Though I was worried about returning quickly, I wouldn't be back again with Jaycee for two years.

ICU Badge Earned: September 2013

It was a simple cold but like so many other times, this cold affected her breathing. I took Jaycee to the emergency room when she seemed to be having some odd combination of symptoms (vomiting, fever, difficulty breathing). By this time in our lives, we had learned to bypass the local hospitals and drive her straight to the children's hospital if we felt it was safe. Not everyone liked this plan, but we turned our van into a "vanbulance." Jaycee had her own pulse oximeter on during the drive, so I could watch her heart rate and oxygen saturation levels. The van's electrical outlet allowed us to do nebulizer treatments on the way if needed. We also had home oxygen tanks ready for these emergencies, which we were able to receive after discussing past problems with our pulmonologist. The van was loaded down with these and other supplies, which was our solution to local hospitals not knowing how to care for Jaycee and wasting precious time.

By: Evana Sandusky

Jason was at work when Jaycee started going downhill that day, so I drafted my mom to be Jaycee's helper in the van on the way. I barked out orders and demanded to know her numbers every few minutes. During our drive, I did have to pull over and put Jaycee on oxygen before resuming to drive as fast as I could to the ER. The oxygen worked at keeping her numbers at a safe place until we arrived.

In the ER, Jaycee tested positive for rhinovirus, which is basically a cold virus. Her X-ray didn't initially look too bad, but her breathing was labored, and she was grunting while breathing, which I had never heard her doing before in these breathing flareups. The oxygen I put on in the van was still needed after we got to the ER. The doctor decided to put her in the ICU as a precaution. It was late at night when the decision was made, so I was just ready for us to be in bed and rest from the tiring day. I was completely exhausted from the stress of the last few hours.

In the ICU, Jaycee was sitting up and watching television right before we settled in for the night. I made her mad when I turned off her movie, as she was ready to party, being hyper from multiple breathing treatments. I told her good night and slept in the chair next to her bed. My mom was resting in a hotel within walking distance from the hospital, since only one of us could stay in Jaycee's room.

A few hours later, a monitor in the room was alarming. I was accustomed to alarms at the hospital, so I didn't respond right away. I figured some probe or sticker came loose, so there was no real danger when the alarm sounded. But when 4-5 people came in talking, watching the monitor, and seemed to be providing some immediate treatment, I surmised something was wrong. I ignorantly asked what the problem was because I didn't see one. Her oxygen saturation levels were in the acceptable range with her asleep on the BiPAP and her heart rate was where it typically runs when she's sick. I wasn't sure what I needed to panic about.

"Her blood pressure is too low to sustain her life" was the answer.

Huh? Her blood pressure? That's never been a problem. I then asked another stupid question, "Should I call my husband?"

Yes, was the resounding answer. My husband, who was driving home from work when we went to the ER, was in contact with me throughout the night. Earlier, I told him everything was fine and not to come over that night. Now, I had to call him and tell him to make the 120-mile trip as fast as he could at three o'clock in the morning.

I watched as a second IV was placed in Jaycee and fluids were pushed in an attempt to raise her pressures. There was a flurry of activity in the room. This type of calm but speedy treatment was new to me, so it was hard to process. The calmness of the healthcare professionals was deceptive. This was nothing like on television where a crisis mode was easy to spot. Everyone was doing his or her job speaking to each other in voices that were firm and focused. Everyone worked quickly, and that is what startled me the most. The doctor working in the ICU that night was extremely nice and relatable. He explained that Jaycee would have to be intubated and have many other things done to her since her body was shutting down for unknown reasons at the time.

I was told I could stay in the room if I wanted. I didn't want to leave Jaycee, but I didn't want to be in the way. People were working all over the room, even removing the headboard for more available space for the pumps and machines they brought in. I left the room as they bagged her in preparation to put her on a ventilator. I'm not sure if I said anything to Jaycee before I left, but I kissed her face, let go of her hand, and felt completely overwhelmed as I stepped out of the room away from my daughter.

I made the short walk to the parents' lounge and sobbed. I didn't understand what was going on. She was stable one minute and near death the next. I called my mom, who was asleep, to come over quickly. For the next few minutes though I was alone.

In the isolation of the lounge, I prayed. It wasn't a deep, spiritual prayer. I was in an exhausted, shocked state. I knew things were serious, but I didn't fully grasp the severity of the situation with everything occurring so rapidly. I prayed that Jaycee would be ok, that the doctors would have wisdom, and that Jaycee wouldn't be scared. I didn't pray long before a thought came to mind: *Jaycee will live.* I knew it wasn't my thought; I knew God was telling me something. Truthfully, I wasn't worried about her not living at that time, but I should have been. I stored that thought away and needed to pull it out several times over the next few weeks as doubt entered.

Soon, my mom joined me in the lounge and sat with me in disbelief. Jason and my father arrived hours later finding us still waiting in the parents' lounge. I had been updated once or twice briefly on Jaycee's condition during the wait; however, I didn't know what questions to ask as this was a new situation. But I did manage to ask the most important one, "Is the worst over?"

The doctor told me it was too soon to tell. His hesitation to answer me helped me understand this was far more severe than anything we had went through with Jaycee.

Finally, much later than we were told, we were escorted back to see Jaycee. Two doctors met us at the door of her room. They explained to us that she was critically ill. They said they were doing everything in their power but couldn't guarantee us that Jaycee would make it through this illness. They asked if we wanted to see the clergy or if there was any family they could call for us. We appreciated the kindness and supportive reactions from the doctors as they explained her condition to us.

I stood listening to them calmly explain Jaycee's condition. I thought back to those times in the ICU when Jaycee was on a BiPAP machine with intubation being threatened. It seemed unimaginable to me, yet here I was thrown into the situation without warning.

I glanced into Jaycee's room and peeked at her monitor. Her oxygen saturation levels were in the upper 80s. I cautiously asked, "Is she on 100% support of the ventilator and her saturations are only in the 80s?"

"Yes. This is serious," they replied.

I knew just how bad it was in that moment. There was no more support they could give her breathing. I cried as I took the scene in fully. Fear immediately came in and tried to attach itself to me. Jason and I walked into the room and looked Jaycee over. She was on numerous IV medications and on a ventilator, which meant she was getting medicine to sedate her. She was also given a drug to paralyze her, so she wouldn't move. She had a catheter to help with bodily fluids and compression pumps on her legs to prevent blood clots as she laid still in bed. She had an arterial line in her wrist to monitor her blood pressure precisely and a central line in her neck. The number of things attached to her was overwhelming. If the speech from the doctors didn't give us cause for concern, one look at her did. We held her hand, prayed over her, and talked to her. We told her, "You are strong, Jaycee. You can beat this. Keep fighting. Keep breathing. You are going to make it." This became our mantra over the next few weeks.

The first 24 hours in the ICU was exhausting. Jaycee was near death, basically in a medically induced coma, so she couldn't even respond to me. It was scary. I didn't want her to die. I prayed and read scriptures to her. Mostly, I tried to hold on to my sanity as it was very difficult to see Jaycee like that and know every second was critical.

Every time the monitor alarmed, I panicked, no longer considering the alarm to be a false beep from a misread. Now every alarm caused me to jump up and look at her numbers. At some point, the beeping and alarming got the best of me and I had a complete breakdown in the parents' lounge. Sometimes, the situation calls for a breakdown; it is inevitable when things are going so wrong.

Things got worse before they got better. The rhinovirus that she tested positive for in the ER was only part of the problem. The doctors informed us her body was in septic shock. Her heart started to fail, along with her lungs. She finally ended up being diagnosed with Acute Respiratory Distress Syndrome (ARDS), which basically meant her lungs were extremely sick. When I Googled the survival rates of those diagnosed with ARDS and septic shock, the numbers were not in our favor, especially given that Jaycee was not a typically healthy child.

Jaycee's illness was intense. As part of the ARDS treatment, she had to be flipped over and placed on her belly, which took a team of people to accomplish given she was on the ventilator and sedated. In general, her body felt the strain of her illness. Her blood pressure would go high and, at other times, alarms would go off for it being too low. Blood pressure medications were added, increased, and decreased. At some point, they place a feeding tube in her. Adjustments were made and remade for her plan of care daily.

For three weeks, we waited, prayed, gave Jaycee pep talks, and watched for any signs of progress. There was hardly a day with complete calmness. When a team of doctors rushed in, we knew it was graver than when just one or two medical professionals visited her room. Each time,

By: Evana Sandusky

I held my breath waiting for the mini-crisis to pass or be treated. I also watched to make sure she was still urinating, as we were told that would be the first sign things were even worse.

During all of this, Jason and I didn't work. We lived at the hospital initially. Jaycee's condition was so bad in the beginning that neither of us wanted to leave her, just in case our worst nightmare happened. We ate, slept, showered, paid bills, and did everything at the hospital. One of us could sleep in her room while the other slept in the parents' lounge; neither was ideal for sleeping. Eventually, we spent a few nights in a hotel a few blocks from the hospital because it was next to impossible to get sleep at the hospital.

The exhaustion of being in the hospital 24 hours a day made it impossible for me to cope with everything that was happening. I now realize that I experienced my first panic attack during this time. I always pictured panic attacks as someone running frantically around, screaming out absurdities, and hyperventilating. I found out those having panic attacks may look just fine on the outside but inside their body is in turmoil. When an alarm sounded and several doctors entered to investigate Jaycee's latest problem, I would immediately get a cold chill, my heart would race, and I worked very hard to control the shaking that my arms and legs instantly did. It usually passed in a few minutes, but it was a frightening sensation that ran through my body. It was uncontrollable and unstoppable. My body was completely stressed. My muscles were so tight, my left arm went numb. My problems weren't the biggest issue at hand, but it is something to note that while Jaycee had care, my husband and I were left to cope on our own.

During all of this, we thought of Elijah often. Elijah was age 4 at the time and stayed with grandma, grandpa, or his aunt while we were in the hospital. He continued attending preschool and tried to maintain a semi-normal routine. We talked on the phone and video chatted a few times, but the video chats seemed to make things worse, as they tended to make him cry when he saw me.

Elijah was able to come visit Jaycee eventually. We debated on whether he should come. He was no stranger to the hospital, but he had never seen his sister on a ventilator. When it became evident that Jaycee wasn't going to come home anytime soon, we decided to let him visit. Our plan was that if he came in the room and seemed upset, we would take him out and never try again. We felt it was important to try. We wanted him to see his sister, whom he loved, and for him to understand we were in the hospital taking care of Jaycee.

The day of the visit came and we watched Elijah closely as he entered. The nurse had covered Jaycee's body up to her neck so that he wouldn't see the wires and lines. She also positioned her head with the ventilator, so it was not the first thing he might see. The nurse did a great job of making Jaycee look more like she was sleeping and less like she was attached to machines all over the room. Elijah was so excited to see his mommy and daddy, and we were excited to see him, too. Elijah is a go with the flow, pay-no-attention-to-the-details kind of kid, so, he was completely fine with the situation. He played with his cars on the windowsill, sat in bed with Jaycee and watched a cartoon, and even kissed her cheek. He was fine, and a good little brother. He spent a few days with us bouncing between the hotel and hospital, and then we had to have a tearful goodbye in the lobby. We did this a few times during her ICU stay. It was a crummy situation to be in as parents, feeling like you must choose which child needs you more in that moment. Neither of us felt we could go home and be with him as it was rare she was completely stable for long periods of time.

Finally, one day Jaycee started to improve. She came down on her ventilator support and passed her trial run that meant she could come off the ventilator completely. She made the switch from the ventilator to the BiPAP on day 21. When she was off the ventilator, she could wake up and move again. There was life in her eyes and it was exciting to see her come back to us. I watched her lifeless form for so long while she was on all the medications that it was a relief to see our Jaycee, the one with some of her personality visible again.

But as she woke up, the toll the illness took on her body became evident to me. While she laid in bed not moving for weeks, her body became very weak. Her already low muscle tone worsened. She couldn't sit up in a chair safely, let alone stand or walk. Physical therapy and occupational therapy were started to help get her skills back. The therapy made me grimace as Jaycee's weak body was made to do things she was no longer capable of doing.

Jaycee only needed a few days on the BiPAP before she was able to step down to oxygen. At that point, she left the intensive care unit. That day was joyful! It meant she didn't require intensive monitoring 24 hours a day and we were one step closer to home. I felt like throwing a party the day Jaycee "graduated" from the ICU. I wanted to leave that room full of awful memories and never return!

On the hospital floor, Jaycee continued to make progress. She acquired enough strength to feed herself though it took her a long time to eat a meal because her hands shook so much from the weakness. It was hard to sit by and watch her struggle to feed herself, but I knew if I did it for her, it would only slow down her progress in the long run. Her therapy continued, and I tried to do little things that I knew would work her muscles. Watching Jaycee for years in physical therapy was paying off.

When Jaycee got off oxygen it became apparent the hospital would not be keeping her just because her skills were diminished from her tone. At that point, Jaycee could feed herself, sit up in bed with pillows surrounding her, and hold a cup. That was about it. If she slouched in her bed, she couldn't get herself out of that position. She couldn't stand safely or walk so going to a bathroom was impossible. She couldn't dress herself either. Jaycee was tired and drugged, too, as she was being weaned off strong medications. She was a much different kid than the one before the hospital. In preparation for going home, I started to try to do all her care without the help of a nurse to see if I could physically do it. Jaycee was extremely weak, and it took all my strength to adjust her in bed or to get her out of the bed and in a chair. She was not a light child; it was easy for my husband to lift her, but not me. I was astounded by her feebleness. I gave her sponge baths, dressed her, and had to learn to change the diaper of a heavy seven-year-old.

When we were close to being discharged, I left Jaycee's room to get some medications from the hospital pharmacy for her. Jaycee was asleep, so it was a good time for me to sneak out. I alerted the nurses that I was leaving Jaycee alone. In the short time I was gone, Jaycee woke up and tried to get out of bed. She didn't realize she couldn't stand or walk on her own yet and a nurse found Jaycee on the floor face down. When I arrived, the nurses and doctor were giving Jaycee a thorough examination to make sure she wasn't hurt from her fall. She was fine, but it showed me how difficult having her at home would be with her low tone and lack of understanding of her situation.

At the end of the fourth week in the hospital, we took Jaycee home. It was exciting but challenging. Jaycee was wheelchair bound and still recovering. We had to add a wheelchair ramp onto the front of the house to have a way to get her into it. My husband and a group of men were nailing in the last board to make the ramp when I arrived home with Jaycee. We made other adjustments, too, like putting her mattress on the floor and using a portable toilet seat to prevent falls. She had about two months of outpatient physical and occupational therapy to gain her skills back. Jaycee couldn't attend school full-time during her recovery, but she did go for a few hours a day, building up the number of days and hours each week.

That time in the ICU can only be described as terrifying and unpredictable. I was grateful Jaycee had survived and lived. It was a miracle actually. I wanted nothing more than to never, ever go through an experience like that again. However, I feared Jaycee would be back again, causing me to earn more ICU Badges.

ICU Badge Earned: August 2014

This badge started with a trip to the dentist. It was innocent enough. Jaycee needed four baby teeth pulled out to give her permanent teeth room to come in her mouth. She was numbed and then given laughing gas for the procedure. Nothing out of the ordinary happened at the dentist. I sat right next to her during the entire procedure, and I was thrilled it was going so well.

On the ride home, Jaycee's mouth was still very numb and she was drooling profusely. As my husband drove home, I sat in the back of the vehicle with Jaycee. For most of the hour-long drive, I had to keep my hand in her mouth to stop her from biting her lip, which was already bleeding and swollen.

When we got home from the dentist, her swollen lip wasn't my only concern. At first, there was a little wheeze that my husband initially swore I was imagining. The next day, Jaycee was still wheezy, and it appeared she was coming down with my son's cold. I was concerned but not to the point of packing for the hospital. Hours later, my concern became real as Jaycee's breathing was wet and congested sounding. To top it off, her oxygen levels were decreasing. Near the end of the day, it was clear, even to my husband, that she needed to go to the emergency room. In less than 24 hours, things went horribly downhill.

Jason drove our "vanbulance" while I monitored Jaycee in the back. By the time we arrived at the ER, Jaycee was on 3 liters of oxygen already. She was immediately taken back for treatment. She tested positive for the rhinovirus again. The x-ray showed a pneumonia that looked like it was aspiration related. It became theorized that Jaycee aspirated while she was leaning back in the dentist chair or while she was numbed and drooling uncontrollably. Jaycee went straight to the ICU as a precaution, but a few hours later her breathing worsened. She went on the BiPAP full-time to support her breathing, as her oxygen saturation levels were dropping in an all too familiar pattern. Her respiratory rate was extremely fast, ranging from 40-60. At one point, her breathing was so labored a group of doctors determined a ventilator may be necessary. They didn't really have to tell us that was a possibility as by that stage of her medical life we knew from the monitors and current interventions that she was headed in that direction. The doctor just confirmed what we were thinking.

My heart sunk. I didn't want to see Jaycee on a ventilator ever again. I didn't want to go through all those emotions and fears and worries. I didn't want to believe Jaycee was *that* sick again. It didn't seem fair for any of us to be in this battle again. Fair or not, we were in it with Jaycee once more.

The doctors decided to try some things like continuous Albuterol to see if it would change her respiratory status and prevent a possible ventilator situation. Over the next few hours, she did better. It wasn't a large change or instantly fixed, but it was a slow pull in the right direction. It took a few days of watching her vital signs slowly improving for the angst of a ventilator became smaller and smaller.

For several days, she was on BiPAP support full-time. During that time, she was so sick that she slept most of the day. When she became more awake she signed for food, but she couldn't eat while she was on support. She would sign: my turn, eat, spaghetti. When I told her she couldn't eat, she would sign a few different signs of hers that indicated she was mad. Nothing about the hospital is easy on a patient or a parent.

Jaycee slowly improved. She was able to be weaned down to a high flow nasal cannula. When she was just on 4 liters of oxygen, she could eat. She was so happy to have a bowl of chicken noodle soup that she ate it in record speed.

On day 8, she left the ICU to go down to the regular hospital floor. On day 10, we were released to go home. I left the hospital with another ICU Badge pinned to me as well as a lot of emotions to sort through from being in this situation again. I also left feeling grateful that Jaycee was leaving the hospital with me to resume our life back home.

Before you read about the next several ICU Badges, I need to share some background information because at some point, you'll probably ask yourself, "Why was this child in the ICU so much?" We had that question ourselves. We asked several doctors about Jaycee's pulmonary issues. We scrutinized their plans and asked for new ideas. Jaycee saw several specialists and tried different or stronger medications. We added new things to our daily routine over the years with little long-term change. Jaycee had bronchoscopies and CT scans of her lungs, which yielded minimal answers. She went through rigorous immunology testing more than once, though we never found a "reason" either. When we felt we weren't getting anywhere with the doctors that Jaycee had seen since she was a toddler, we looked elsewhere.

We ended up pursuing a second opinion from a reputable hospital over three hours from our house. Jaycee was examined by several specialists there and had more scans and another bronchoscopy, complete with washes and biopsies. Jaycee had this medical test and that one. Small findings, like GERD, were discovered in this process, but there was never a major diagnosis or reason given for her respiratory issues. More medications were added in hopes of helping her, but a real solution to these admissions was never found. We had hoped for a long time that simple changes or new medications would keep Jaycee from getting so sick but that hope was always crushed by an illness that attacked her body and sent her to the emergency room.

As you continue reading this chapter, please remember that we tried to look for answers. We sought out experts. We tried to get our daughter help, but if there is no diagnosable condition found, then there can be no real treatment to prevent further admissions. We still don't have good answers for Jaycee's respiratory issues, and perhaps, we never will.

ICU Badge Earned: June 2015

Jaycee made it 9 months without a hospital admission. I was feeling great about her health. The longer she stayed healthy, the better off she'd be if an illness ever arose. At least, that was my thought process but, sadly, I was wrong.

This illness, like so many others, started off with a cough. Her lungs sounded like they were full of mucus which immediately sent me into a heightened state of administering home medications and frequent monitoring. Just thirty-six hours later we headed off to the emergency room after Jaycee's oxygen saturations started to drop when she was sleeping.

Even though it was the middle of the night, I must admit that Jaycee didn't look as ill as she had in the past. Her vital signs on arrival weren't too worrisome and because of that, we were being ignored by the night ER staff. The first doctor went over her symptoms, commented that she looked well, and ordered a chest X-ray. No nurse checked on her, no one hooked her up to any kind of monitors—it wasn't the type of emergency room experience we were accustomed to receiving. I suppose they didn't believe us when we reported numbers in the low 80s while she slept with her CPAP on at home. After hours of sitting in a small room with no medical intervention being provided and no monitoring being done, my husband and I were beyond frustrated.

The next time we saw the doctor he reported her X-ray looked like a viral infection. He heroically announced that Jaycee could go home if we were comfortable. Obviously, we weren't comfortable or we wouldn't have come in the middle of the night to a hospital two hours away. Besides, the chest X-ray and vitals were taken at triage hours ago, while nothing had been completed by the ER department. How could they even tell if she was well enough to go home? We voiced our concerns and the doctor left to get the attending doctor. When he exited, I begged my husband to be assertive with the next doctor and demand something be done. He had already planned to do whatever was necessary to get Jaycee help, so I really didn't have to plead with him at all.

The attending doctor came in with his opinion of Jaycee before he heard our concerns. He updated us and sounded as if he was going to discharge Jaycee. That's when my husband spoke about his worries for Jaycee and annoyance over her lack of care thus far. The doctor insisted Jaycee wasn't that bad but humored us by putting on the oxygen saturation monitor.

It was no surprise to me that it showed her oxygen saturations were bouncing around and dipping into the mid-80s. The doctor began to change his opinion of Jaycee and decided the hospital was where she needed to stay. Finally, she was thoroughly checked over, a nurse made a first appearance, and a breathing treatment was ordered *five hours* after arriving. Eventually, an oxygen cannula was placed on Jaycee, too. This all took place at the hospital we trusted. I excused myself from the room and went into the bathroom and cried. I was so exasperated! It is so terrible to know something is wrong with your child and to be ignored—again and again. After multiple hospital admissions, one would think the ER physicians would take our concerns seriously, but it wasn't the case. It's vexing when you are not heard and are considered paranoid. This situation is why I hate going to the ER. I never know what sort of treatment my child will receive and if I will find myself in a situation fighting for Jaycee's care. I know Jaycee though; her numbers can look fine and then drop dramatically without warning. We weren't upset over nothing! After those bottled-up emotions came out, I rejoined Jaycee in the emergency room, relieved she was going to be admitted and get the care she needed.

When she finally got into her room on the pulmonary floor of the hospital, we were all ready to go to sleep after being awake all night long and being stressed for several hours. I pulled up my chair next to Jaycee's bed and was prepared to sleep sitting up for the next few hours as my husband crashed on the one couch in the room. When Jaycee drifted off to sleep, her oxygen support increased substantially to the point that the rapid response team had to be called. I had gotten only minutes of sleep when adrenaline kicked in as I tried to process the change of status.

By: Evana Sandusky

A couple of hours ago, the ER doctor was on the verge of discharging us. Now, Jaycee was going to the Intensive Care Unit to be placed on continuous BiPAP support—again. I was still in disbelief when I sat by Jaycee's ICU bed trying not to think about what would have happened if we had gone home. Thank God that doctor took a second look at her after my husband spoke up! But what about all that wasted time? Could some of it had been prevented if they had started interventions sooner?

Two days later, Jaycee's breathing was much worse. Rhinovirus and pneumonia were the main problems once again. Jaycee's respiratory rate kept getting faster and faster. The support she needed on the BiPAP kept increasing; Jaycee was not doing well. I didn't need anyone to tell me what would come next because I knew. That's the one helpful thing about being in the ICU more than once—you know what to expect. One night things kept getting worse with Jaycee. My exhausted husband, who was sick with the same cold at the time, was getting rest at a nearby hotel. I was up half of the night watching the monitor, praying for a miracle, and coming to terms with the possibility that a ventilator may happen. I didn't want a ventilator. I didn't want Jaycee to go through all that again, especially not at 9-years old. To be honest, I didn't want to live through it again. I prayed against the ventilator and prayed harder for a miracle. Then my friend messaged me in the wee hours of the morning. She sent me a scripture and a lovely word of encouragement. God was gracious to send me a word through my friend, Amanda. I didn't need to fear a ventilator if that was what Jaycee needed. I didn't need to let my trepidations run wild. I accepted the possibility a ventilator might happen, and I was finally ready to think logically. When Jason came back the following day the ICU team discussed options with us at morning rounds. Our first possibility was to keep Jaycee on her BiPAP, accept oxygen saturation levels in the 80s, and see what happens; going this route would require a ventilator be put on in a rush when her levels got too low for too long. Option two was to put Jaycee on the ventilator as a pre-emptive strike to allow her lungs to rest and heal. I knew Jaycee—she wasn't going to get magically better on her own at this point. In the long run, we decided to put her on the ventilator in her present state instead of waiting for her condition to worsen and have an emergent situation.

After Jaycee's ordeal with the ventilator in 2013, I must admit Jaycee being on a ventilator due to a respiratory illness again was probably my biggest fear. Yet there we were suddenly in the exact same nightmare. The first time I saw Jaycee with that tube down her throat, the arterial line stitched into her wrist, the urine catheter taped to her leg, the PICC line in her arm, and two more IV lines in her body, was overwhelming. There was no denying she was sick again and needed the necessary apparatus, no matter how much I despised them. Knowing my daughter, who had been healthy for nine months, was once again fighting for her life in the ICU became unbearable. The tears came rolling out as thoughts whirled in my mind.

Life in ICU isn't easy, even after acquiring several ICU Badges. There is never a boring or calm time with an ICU Badge. Outside, life moves on, even when it seems to stop for you in the hospital. My husband celebrated Father's Day that year holding Jaycee's hand while she was sedated on the ventilator. It was a Father's Day that neither of us will forget, but we would certainly like to. We also canceled a camping trip that we had planned to Branson; a trip we had all been excited about. Luckily, we made it to Branson later that year in December.

Jaycee spent the next several days going up and down on her support on the ventilator. One moment, I felt she was making progress but then something happened out of nowhere that slammed me back into the cruel unpredictable world of ICU. Her blood pressure frequently alarmed for being too low, jarring me day and night. Medications were also needed to treat different responses her body was having to the illness. Eventually, an NG tube was placed since she couldn't eat by mouth. In rounds, the doctors used the technical terms to describe what I saw right in front of me. "Respiratory failure" was said so causally in rounds that I felt strangely calm when it was listed as a diagnosis.

Finally, the morning came for the ventilator to be taken off. I was cautiously excited and did something you never do when a big event is going to happen. I told people the ventilator was coming off through Jaycee's Caring Bridge website. That was a rookie mistake. I knew better than to tell people what *was* going to happen on her site. I usually only reported what *has* happened, since things change quickly in a hospital. A few hours after my happy announcement, I had to backtrack and report that it wasn't happening that day. Jaycee's breathing deteriorated and needed more support, so it stayed on for another day.

The next day we were all joyous as Jaycee was able to be transitioned to the BiPAP machine once again. Jaycee spent a total of 10 days on the ventilator, and it was great to see her without that tube hanging out of her mouth. It meant she was on the road to recovery. Jaycee was still too sick to eat or drink but frequently asked for pizza, spaghetti, and mashed potatoes in sign language. I loved when she communicated with me, and clearly food consumed her thoughts when she was deprived of it. I'm sure I'd be the same way in that situation.

In a few days, she was on a nasal cannula and ready to move hospital floors. Leaving the ICU with Jaycee that time brought me so much happiness. I felt like she was walking across the stage at a graduation, except it was Jaycee being pushed in a wheelchair down the hall and out of the doors of the ICU. Familiar nurses happily waved goodbye to Jaycee and told her not to come back. Some of these nurses were the same ones who cared for Jaycee during her scary septic shock and ARDS admission in 2013. They each recalled how Jaycee gave them a good scare that admission, and I was surprised at how many people remembered that illness and our family.

After a total of three weeks, Jaycee was able to be pushed out the front door of the hospital and taken back home. Three weeks! And it all started with a doctor who almost sent her home.

Another ICU Badge was firmly fixed onto me with hope there wouldn't be more. How many times can one little child have so many serious illnesses? I was starting to feel a bit traumatized by all these ICU stays. I wasn't sure how to cope with a life that regularly involved the ICU. It was never easy on anyone in our family but most of all Jaycee.

ICU Badge Earned: October 2015

After Jaycee's rough summer illness on the ventilator, I was worried the fall would bring trouble. August and September are notoriously bad months for Jaycee's breathing. We live in a rural area with fall foliage, farmers harvesting their corn and bean crops, and dusty gravel roads. Add in the start of school with increased germ exposure and humid, hot air, and it's a perfect storm for an asthmatic. When those months came and went, we all breathed a sigh of relief. Jaycee had made it through the first part of school without an absence for an illness. Then, once again, life was interrupted with a cough. Breathing treatments were started at home and a visit to the doctor was scheduled. Oral steroids were started for her one and only symptom, a cough that produced mucus.

If you have read the preceding stories, you can probably predict how this ICU Badge was earned. This time the visit to the ER at one in the morning went off without any issues from the staff. A chest X-ray indicated pneumonia in the bases of both lungs. An IV was placed, medication was given, and her oxygen requirement was pushed to 8 liters in the ER before the BiPAP machine made its way into the room. In just two hours, all of this was completed, and Jaycee was on her way to the ICU. Two hours in the ER is a very short time. I was glad this experience was going better than our previous one.

Jaycee had a few hiccups with her blood pressure and breathing, but she was out of ICU on day four. And on day six, Jaycee was back at home. This ICU Badge was given for a time that was relatively calm after a rocky start. If there is something to be thankful for when earning badges that don't want to be earned, it is that this one was a short stay.

ICU Badge Earned: May 2016

Seven months. That is how long Jaycee had gone without a hospital admission. She had a couple of illnesses, which were successfully treated at home, but Jaycee's health was great, so I was not too worried when I saw the first signs of a cold developing. I started Jaycee's yellow zone asthma medications as soon as I saw snot and heard her cough.

If there ever was a time to be sick, this was not the time for it! After spending thirteen years in the same home, we were moving to a new home just a few miles away. During our move, Jaycee's

By: Evana Sandusky

grandfather watched her and gave her medications every few hours as the rest of our family loaded up all our belongings and helped us settle in to our new home.

While I continued to unpack items and figure out where to store things in the new home over the next few days, Jaycee's cold persisted. I continued treating her at home and monitoring her closely. On the fourth night in the new house, I woke up at two o'clock in the morning because the light in our master bathroom was on. I reached over to pat the bed, making sure my husband was the one in the bathroom, but I ended up hitting Jason's chest.

In the moment between being awake and asleep, I calmly asked my husband, "Who's in our bathroom?"

He got up to check, since he was more awake from my slap to his chest, and announced Jaycee was using the bathroom, and everything was fine.

After a few minutes, my eyes were fully opened, and I made my way towards the bathroom to see for myself. Jaycee being up in the middle of the night while she had a cold was an usually bad sign.

There it was. The scene I had been dreading for months. My daughter had blue lips and toes. "Jason, she's blue!" I exclaimed as I raced to the rescue inhalers.

My husband and I sprang into our emergency mode. We had done this many times, so we knew the process instinctively. One of us grabbed the thermometer—she had a fever. One of us hooked her up to her monitor—low saturations. Medication was given. The time was noted so we could repeat the steps again in 20 minutes. Tylenol was given and a plastic tub to catch the impending vomiting was placed nearby.

Soon, Jaycee was loaded into the van with all our supplies and monitors. I drove her to the emergency room alone, since my husband had just gotten into bed after working late. The local emergency room did well. I rarely used a local emergency room anymore because of past experiences. By the time I arrived at the emergency room, Jaycee's breathing was no longer labored. I was pretty sure they would check her over and send us home with medications.

Over the course of the next few hours sitting in the emergency room, all that had changed. Her breathing started to become more labored. The doctors and nurses were very responsive to Jaycee and for that I was happy I had chosen this emergency room. After the pediatrician assessed Jaycee, she determined Jaycee needed to be transferred to the children's hospital and given continuous Albuterol while waiting for the ambulance to arrive.

When the transport team arrived hours later, they decided Jaycee didn't need the continuous Albuterol, which had miraculously helped her breathing. That would prove later to be a big mistake. From their perspective, she didn't look like she needed it, but they hadn't seen Jaycee in the previous state a few hours earlier.

With Jason at work, I drove to the next emergency room where Jaycee and I would wait for the next few hours. Clearly, Jaycee needed to be admitted, no one was denying that. The holdup was deciding if Jaycee needed to be admitted to the pulmonary floor or the ICU.

 The doctors were fine monitoring her and even stopped the breathing treatments to see how long she could go without needing one. Finally, it became evident Jaycee needed support that only the ICU could provide.

As far as hospital stays go, this one was calm in one respect. There were no emergencies where doctors suddenly filled the room. Jaycee made slow progress as she was first weaned from her BiPAP and then from continuous Albuterol and later off oxygen altogether.

There was one issue that came up during this stay that I would rather forget. On Jaycee's first full day in the ICU, I was taken into a room and questioned by a social worker. Social worker visits were normal in the hospital as they offer help in a variety of ways. But, the supportive tone of the typical encounters was not present this time.

I was taken to a conference room down the hall from my child when the typical questions started. Suddenly, it launched into questions about Jaycee's daily care. I recited her medicines from memory. The social worker marveled that I could work and keep track of all of Jaycee's needs and appointments.

Then the questions were directed to the present illness. When did I take her to the doctor? Why didn't I take her back when she got worse? Did I give her this or that rescue medication? Did

I try this at home? Why didn't I call the on-call pulmonologist? Where was my husband? My daughter was in ICU, but I didn't seem very upset about it. Was I aware of how sick she was?

This was a **long** conversation. By the end of it, I was convinced the social worker was going to make a hotline call to report me for negligent parenting (Thankfully, it never happened.). Had Jaycee's X-ray showed pneumonia, this conversation wouldn't have happened. But, because she merely had an asthmatic reaction to a virus, my parenting was called into question. I called a few of my friends and Jaycee's teachers to prepare them to be character witnesses for me, if the need came, because I was truly afraid of what this woman would do.

I felt like my favorite "Seinfeld" character, George Costanza. I thought of a million comebacks and things I should have said after the conversation. These included: *Maybe if your ER hadn't stopped the continuous Albuterol that the first ER started that helped her, then maybe she would be fine now. And maybe if your ER hadn't let her go hours without a breathing treatment to "see how she would do," she may be in a better spot right now. Jaycee is prone to getting sick quickly, and if you look at her chart, you'll see she has a complicated history that I can't help.*

But, I didn't say any of it. Frankly, I had been up for about 30 hours with almost no sleep before this conversation and wasn't thinking sharply. I was so upset by the tone of the conversation after spending the days before the hospital admission monitoring my daughter, giving her medications, literally pacing the floors, and stressing myself out over her illness. I didn't want her to be in the hospital, but her lungs weren't strong nor healthy.

Jaycee spent five nights in the hospital for this illness, which was determined to be an asthma exacerbation due to rhinovirus. I wanted her recovery to go quickly so I could get away from a medical establishment that I now felt wasn't on our side. Before Jaycee was discharged, the social worker dropped by her room again to remind me to be vigilant with Jaycee's care next time. I took that as a warning.

When we loaded up into the van to finally make the trip home, Jaycee and I were both happy this hospital stay was over. We celebrated by eating Chick-fil-A on the way, and I made room on my sash for yet another badge. This one was heavy though because it called into question my care-taking abilities. Once again, I was portrayed as a horrible mother.

For weeks, I replayed the conversation with the social worker in my head. I questioned my decisions and actions, cried, and cried some more. I tortured myself when I knew, deep down, I was not responsible for Jaycee's hospital stay. My husband was furious with what had been said to me at the hospital. He knows how anxious I get at home when Jaycee is sick; plus, he knows I did everything to help her. I felt further vindicated when I discussed this later with Jaycee's primary care physician, who was quite angry someone had the crudeness to have such a conversation with me. I let go of some of my self-blame after that and prayed that Jaycee would stay healthy for a very long time. Thankfully, it would be over a year later before we would see the ICU again, and I wouldn't see that social worker the next time!

ICU Badge Earned: November 2017

It was the night before Thanksgiving, and nothing was out of the ordinary. I was preparing some desserts for the feast the next day, the kids were watching movies—everything was completely normal when we put Jaycee to bed.

About an hour later, Jaycee came out of her room crying. This was highly unusual. The next hour was spent trying to figure out what was wrong with her. She was vomiting, running a fever, and seemed to be in pain. Her breathing seemed fast, but it was hard to decipher what was going on. When we put her to bed, she was not sick in any way. Now, our minimally verbal child was unable to tell us what was wrong.

Finally, I decided to take Jaycee to the emergency room. Her color didn't seem right. I was concerned about her breathing, but our home monitor was having a hard time reading on her very cold hands. Before we left, we made a call to grandpa who lived a minute away to come sleep at the house with Elijah while we both went to the ER with Jaycee.

When we arrived, we were happy to see it wasn't busy at all. Jaycee was taken right back and evaluated. The doctors were concerned with her immediately because her heart rate was elevated

By: Evana Sandusky

and her blood pressure kept trending towards the low side. Her vomiting continued with the addition of diarrhea, which was a problem I had not come prepared to deal with in the ER. I ran out of wipes and extra clothes quickly. A chest X-ray showed pneumonia. It was hard to believe she developed pneumonia when her symptoms went from mild to serious in hours, not days. Not long after being there, they decided Jaycee needed to be transferred to the St. Louis Children's Hospital. While we waited for the ambulance to arrive, oxygen was placed on Jaycee.

Jason decided to go home, get a few hours of sleep, and pack for an extended hospital stay. Meanwhile, I waited until the early hours of the morning for the ambulance and caught a ride with it to the hospital.

At the Children's Hospital, Jaycee's vital signs continued to worsen in their emergency room. To stabilize her blood pressure, bags of IV fluids were pushed. As people were waking up to celebrate Thanksgiving Day, I had already endured a marathon night with Jaycee and was now in the ICU.

Later that morning, Jason brought Elijah to the hospital, so we could be together for the holiday. We spent time in Jaycee's room watching movies and listening to her breathe via a continuous CPAP machine. Because food wasn't allowed her in ICU room, we ate in shifts. Jason ate alone in the cafeteria, which was serving their version of a turkey dinner. I ate with Elijah right afterwards. I was sad we were celebrating a holiday in the hospital, but at the same time, I knew other families had been there for weeks and months. I would miss seeing my family today and the Black Friday shopping tomorrow, but the most important thing was Jaycee's health.

I guess if there's a positive aspect about her getting sick, it was that it occurred at a "good" time. My husband, who had just started a new job about eight weeks prior, just happened to be home for the holiday. Elijah was able to stay with his dad in a nearby hotel for a couple of days since he was off from work. It was nice having the family together, even if it was in the hospital. Jason was scheduled to go to a job in another state hours away on the Monday after Thanksgiving. Fortunately, his work gave him some extra time off while Jaycee was in the hospital. There's a part of me that wants to believe that there's nothing good about the hospital, but a few things worked this time.

Breathing, as usual, was her main problem. For four days, Jaycee relied on the CPAP to give her breath. She couldn't eat or drink during that time because of the risk of aspiration. Jaycee didn't feel well. She was sad and easily agitated when the nurses tried to care for her. Jaycee took comfort in her favorite movie, *Beauty and the Beast*. The staff noticed that it was on nearly all the time. As soon as the credits started, she would push replay on her iPad.

On the fifth day, Jaycee finally made some progress with her breathing and made the switch from CPAP to high flow nasal cannula. Less oxygen support meant she could at least drink something. She asked for "spaghetti" in sign language repeatedly, however, the doctor told her no.

After Jaycee drifted off to sleep that night, Jason and I decided to leave the hospital for some good old-fashioned stress eating. However, when I saw the van in the parking garage, I immediately noticed someone had stolen the registration sticker off my license plate. I was furious. I had a complete meltdown in the parking lot. It wasn't so much about the sticker but the culmination of everything. It seemed very pathetic that someone would steal from a vehicle in a hospital parking garage. I needed a double order for my stress eating after that discovery.

My anger subsided by the next day, though I still whined to several hospital staff who were willing to listen to me. I had a reason to be happy on this day though because Christmas was kicking off at the hospital. All of the Christmas lights were being turned on at an official ceremony. Christmas cookies were given to the parents. Free things were rare at the hospital, so this was a real treat! Special visitors made rounds throughout the hospital to see the patients. Santa stood outside of Jaycee's ICU room and gave her a wave and blew her a kiss since Jaycee was on isolation, Santa couldn't come inside her room. Jaycee enjoyed his short visit, nevertheless. She pointed to him and gave a little smile while receiving breath from the high flow nasal cannula. Santa even left Jaycee some incredible gifts.

Within the next couple of days, Jaycee was doing well enough to be moved out of ICU. She was so excited when she was able to have spaghetti and pizza. She devoured those first foods, and I was happy she could do something she wanted.

When we went home on day 10, I had another badge on my sash and another reason to be grateful for my daughter's life.

The collection of ICU Badges has been the hardest and most unexpected ones I have collected. Each badge represents a nightmare and a miracle all in one. These badges have shaped me the most as a parent, since I know that tomorrow isn't guaranteed. They remind me that every healthy day with my children is a blessing. These badges give me an outlook on life that many people don't have because they haven't experienced these situations with their child. I know what's important in life.

On the other hand, these badges have taken a significant toll on me. I experienced anxiety, stress, and fear like nothing else in my life. I have cried, worried myself sick, and became angry over health scares I could not control. I have woken up in a panic from hospital related nightmares in the dead of night and had to convince myself that Jaycee and I were both safe at home. Those dreams felt so real that I relived scenes again and again well after the danger was over. I have bottled up stress and anxiety from hospital stays to the point I have questioned my own sanity at times and wondered if I could endure anymore heartache with my child. These badges haven't been easy as a mother. They certainly haven't been easy on Jaycee, who is enduring far worse than I ever could imagine.

I never pictured myself adorning so many ICU Badges for caring for my sweet daughter in such a scary and unpredictable place. I pray that I have supported Jaycee well through it all because she is the main person bearing the extent of the pain.

By: Evana Sandusky

CHAPTER 5:

THE HOME MEDICAL BADGE

Home Medical Badge: This badge is earned when a mom must provide medical interventions at home to keep her child healthy. This includes necessary prescription medications or specialized medical equipment. This badge is only earned once, but training and experience associated with this badge may vary from mom to mom.

Home Medical Badge Earned: 2006

My Home Medical Badge was earned the moment we brought Jaycee home from the hospital. Jaycee was on a few different medications for congestive heart failure. I remember feeling so odd that syringes and medication bottles were a vital part of my newborn's daily routine. I worried about forgetting a medicine or missing a dose. I felt pressure to make sure I did things correctly because her tiny body was depending on me to get it right.

It was a monumental task, at times, getting Jaycee to keep down the medicines, as she had a strong gag reflex and acid reflux. It was so frustrating when she would spit out a medication because if I redrew the medicine, then we would run out early and I would not know exactly how much she ingested. I had to learn how to ease the medications in her mouth, so she would keep it down. I also learned how to hide medicines in liquids or nipples to get her to take them. Things eventually got easier, and Jaycee became accustomed to medication.

Now that Jaycee has gotten older, I have become more adapted to giving medications, as they are still a part of her daily life. I don't worry about forgetting a medicine as much now; my brain is programmed to dish out prescriptions two times a day without thinking about it. There are only a few medicines that Jaycee doesn't take well, but for the most part, she will swallow them without any problems. Jaycee knows what medications she takes and when she takes them. If her routine is maintained, she is accepting of the medication. When she is sick and more medications are added, she knows something is wrong and tends to spit those medications out. In a way, I'm still struggling with similar issues from when Jaycee first came home. Many years later, syringes and medication bottles are still necessary items in our house.

Besides oral medication, a nebulizer was started at an early age. The nebulizer, and all its associated parts, took a place in our home permanently in 2006. This was something that felt foreign at first, too. Medication through a syringe took relatively little time whereas a nebulizer treatment required some forethought and planning. Sitting with her on the couch for 15 minutes or so daily letting the medication dispense was a change to our daily routine.

Jaycee tolerated the nebulizer treatments well, but it was hard for me to accept that my child needed another medical intervention to stay healthy. With every addition to our routine, I found it took me a few weeks (or sometimes longer) to fully adjust to the change. Jaycee usually adjusted quicker than I did.

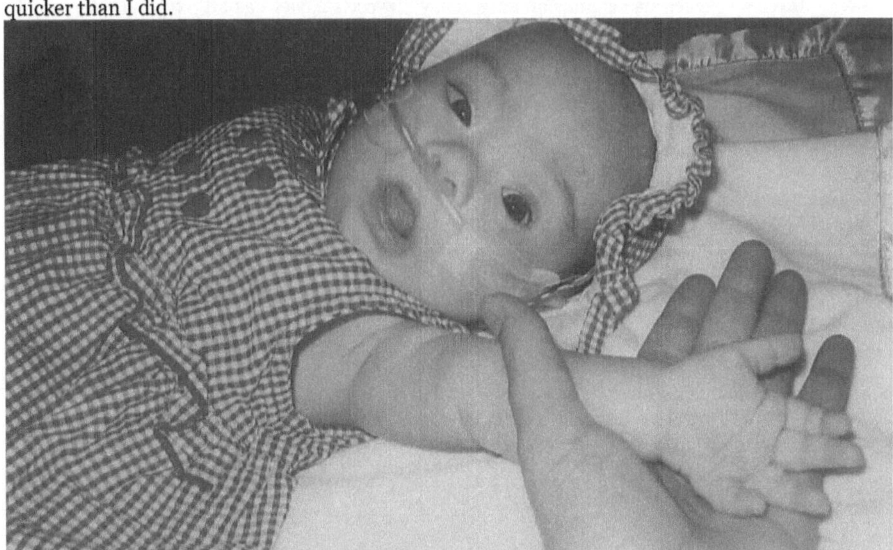

Jaycee on Home Oxygen in 2006

Oxygen tanks were added to my badge experience after Jaycee's first heart surgery. For three months, I carried my baby around attached to a small oxygen tank. Because she was only 3-6 months old while she was on oxygen, I had to make sure Jaycee didn't unintentionally pull off her oxygen cannula. This meant I had to tape the cannula on as securely as possible with hopes of minimal irritation to her face. It was interesting when I had to do this by myself because a baby just doesn't lay still. During her sleep, I found myself checking on her to make sure she hadn't rolled on top of her oxygen line or pinched it off somehow. I worried about her, especially as she got more active.

Life with an oxygen tube felt like life with a leash at times. She was tied to the oxygen tank and could only go so far with it. If I had to change her diaper, then picking her up and moving her to the changing table while rolling her tank behind us became a much more difficult task than it needed to be. Instead, I changed her diaper wherever she was when the time came. For bathing, I used a portable infant bathtub in the living room where I had more room to maneuver her and the tank. I felt the oxygen tank was limiting her experiences in the world since moving her and the tank felt awkward until time and practice helped me feel more comfortable.

Going out with the oxygen tank was obstinate, too. Picture me carrying Jaycee in the infant car seat with the portable oxygen tank bag draped on one shoulder while lugging a diaper bag on the other shoulder. It wasn't easy, and I hated that my baby needed so much stuff for an outing or appointment. Then there were those awkward moments when we were dining out and someone would light a cigarette near us. We would have to leave the restaurant or ask for another seat. (Thankfully, smoking bans in my state have eliminated that problem now.) I was so happy when the oxygen tanks left our house at the end of her recovery. It was a great day. I thought we would part forever.

However, the oxygen tanks came back in the house when Jaycee was about six years old. By that time, Jaycee had turned blue from respiratory distress at our home several times, resulting in expensive trips to the emergency room. It was decided that home oxygen was necessary to have on stand-by in order for us to give Jaycee immediate care and get her to the hospital safely.

By: Evana Sandusky

Now Jaycee's oxygen use signals an emergency. Jaycee's closet has an oxygen tank ready to go, complete with a nasal cannula attached to it with all the necessary items needed. It's a different experience with oxygen than we had years ago, and a much more urgent situation, but also one that we have experienced so many times that it seems familiar.

When Jaycee has trouble breathing now, we sometimes must put the oxygen on before we leave for the emergency room. Sometimes, we start heading to the hospital and must pull over to put on the oxygen. Other times, we get to the hospital before we ever need it. The home oxygen tank is just one of those things that we are glad to have around the house when we need it, but we hope we never need it often.

The Home Medical Badge experience continued when Jaycee started using a CPAP and later a BiPAP machine. The CPAP was by far the hardest piece of medical equipment that was added to our daily routine. Jaycee was young and didn't understand why she had to wear this strange contraption on her face. I had little support from the medical professionals on how to best introduce the machine to get her accustomed to it. It felt like they were insinuating, "Here's her machine, she needs to wear it, or she can't breathe well at night. Good luck." Talk about pressure!

The biggest obstacle with the CPAP was Jaycee did not tolerate it well. She didn't like the mask, which seemed flimsy and not made securely enough for a small child. Jaycee was a wild sleeper who flipped and flopped all night long. The mask had no chance of staying on perfectly during sleep that involved so much movement. Sometimes, the mask slipped off but other times, I know she took it off. I really can't blame her; she didn't understand its importance.

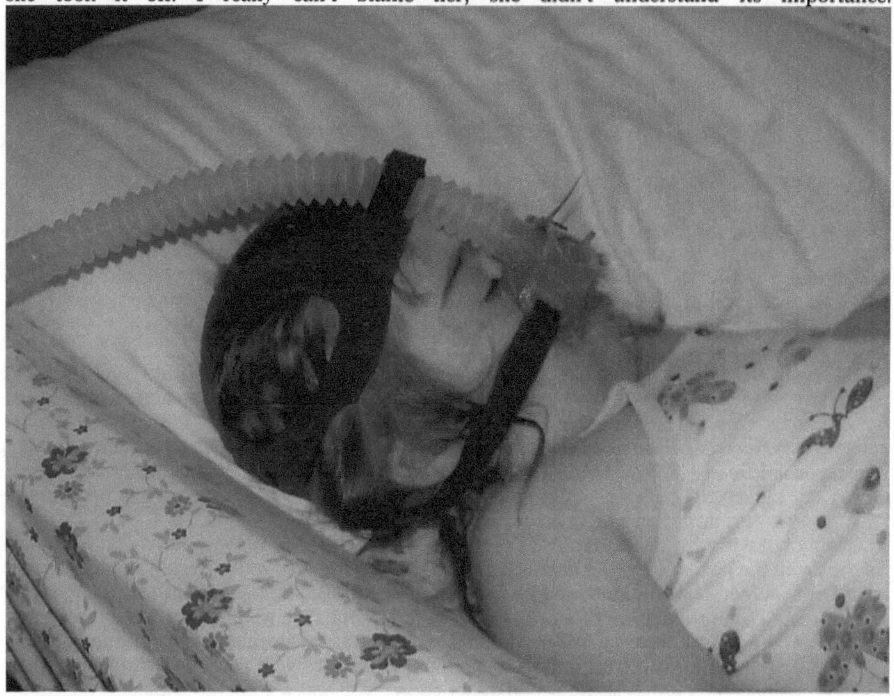

Jaycee on her CPAP Mask that We Struggled with for Years

Still, I was persistent. I kept trying every night even though she never wore it a full night. The severity of her sleep apnea scared me, so I felt personally responsible. Even though I wanted to give up, I kept trying. Unfortunately, there weren't too many other cases of children wearing CPAP machines; according to our local medical supplier, Jaycee was only 1 of 2 children in the area they served that used one. So, they didn't have any good advice for me. Doctors and nurses described Jaycee's inability to wear it as a "behavioral problem," stating she must be "stubborn" or "defiant" about her mask. I didn't see it that way at all and was quite irritated. I received tons of bad advice from people who seemed to forget she was a three-year-old, non-verbal child with Down syndrome that had limited understanding.

I was told to make her wear the mask and push past her defiance. All the while, I complained about her poorly constructed mask and asked for a different mask and headgear to try instead. There surely had to be something that would stay in place better and be more comfortable for her. These complaints seemed to fall on deaf ears though.

Every time I walked into Jaycee's room with that mask laying on the floor instead of on her face, I just wanted to scream. I was mad and frustrated at the situation and lack of support. It was awful to keep putting it on her even though she hated it. I was mad at multiple attempts to put the mask on her each night with seemingly no improvement. I was aggravated surgery didn't fix her obstructive sleep apnea. I hated that CPAP machine and dreaded nighttime, as my nights were no longer peaceful, nor were Jaycee's. I struggled emotionally for months trying to make this equipment "work."

Every night for years, it was the same battle. I waited for Jaycee to fall asleep to start the game of on again-off again with the mask. Eventually, I found more success by putting it on her after 20 minutes or so of sleep, so she wouldn't immediately want to take it off. Then I would check on her a few times before going to bed myself. Usually, the mask was off or partially off during these checks, which meant I had to put it on her again.

Waiting for Jaycee to fall asleep to start the process was sometimes exhausting itself. When she was three, she had a regular bedtime, but her sleep time was inconsistent. Sometimes, she went right to sleep, other times she would be awake until 11 pm, which meant I was up beyond 11 pm. On nights when we had a late outing, it made it even later for both us to go to sleep.

All of this was a major adjustment for me. I didn't have a good attitude about it since nothing about it seemed to be working. I needed support from her medical team, and there was none. I would have given up but the fear of her stopping breathing during her sleep pushed me through those hard times. I just wanted Jaycee to sleep safely. What was the point of all those tests and getting equipment if there was no support for the child at home?

The CPAP changed Jaycee's childhood in another way, too. Jaycee could not have a spontaneous sleepover with grandma, or anyone else for that matter. She had to go home instead. It seemed unjust for Jaycee who couldn't just stay with her cousins if they were having fun one evening. Planned sleepovers were few for her since spending the night required me to transport her machine and teach that person how to put it on and use it. Even as Jaycee has aged, she has only ever stayed the night with her grandparents, who have some familiarity with a CPAP since grandpa uses one, too.

Sometimes, it was hard seeing Jaycee's childhood so different because of this medical need. Early on, I was hopeful Jaycee would one day outgrow her sleep apnea. I didn't want to have to position her bed next to an outlet for her machine to use for the rest of her life or worry about moving her into her bedroom if she fell asleep on the couch. I didn't want to have to worry about the long-term effects on her lungs and heart from the apneic events either. For all these reasons, I prayed for her to outgrow this problem, hoping the sleep study reports would show improvement, even though I knew the chances were slim. I suppose I couldn't handle the finality of the machine coming into our house. Thinking the machine was temporary was perhaps a coping mechanism. At this point, I'm doubtful her obstructive sleep apnea will ever just go away, and so are the doctors. Now, I pray her obstructive sleep apnea will not become more severe.

I was wrong again. A change in Jaycee's severity ended our time with the CPAP, but a BiPAP machine took its place. The hope was for Jaycee to tolerate the higher-pressure settings better. Around that same time, I met a sleep lab technician during a sleep study who introduced me to a mask that covered her face totally (eyes, nose, and mouth). It was the mask I was dreaming about! This mask had a secure fit and wouldn't slip when she flopped around at night. I couldn't believe this mask existed, especially when I had been asking for years about a different mask!

By: Evana Sandusky

Things changed when these two items were started. Jaycee kept wearing the BiPAP for longer periods of time, which meant I didn't have to reposition the mask every time I walked by her bedroom at night. The scuba-looking face mask was the solution we needed! Finally, at age 7 Jaycee was wearing the mask all night long without any problems—almost four (long) years for her to fully adjust to the machine treating her sleep apnea! It was awesome! She eventually tolerated the mask going on her when she was put to bed too, which was another huge milestone.

The BiPAP has taken a permanent spot in our home while expanding my home medical equipment knowledge. I have come to a place where her machine use at night is just another step in our day like brushing teeth or taking a shower. There's not really any good or bad emotions tied to it, it's just something I do for Jaycee. The anger I once felt is all gone, but the situation is finally better. I'm grateful she tolerates her mask and machine now, so she can breathe at night. We are both sleeping better now.

If the CPAP was the piece of medical equipment that I hated the most, the oxygen saturation monitor was the exact opposite. I welcomed this piece of equipment into our home with open arms. With Jaycee's obstructive sleep apnea and her frequent illnesses, I needed a home oxygen saturation monitor to better care for her. Prior to the monitor, I had a hard time discerning whether Jaycee just sounded like she was breathing poorly or if she really was having difficulty breathing. I would examine her lips and fingers to determine if there was a hint of a blue hue to them, but I hated the fact I had to rely on my untrained eyes and ears. I would sometimes call family over to the house to ask if they thought her color seemed odd or not. Of course, I took her to the doctor too, but I worried at home by myself.

Usually, I was told I was being paranoid. Jaycee, being nonverbal, couldn't communicate anything about an illness or pain. I had to read into every action or lack of reaction to try to guess what was going on with her body. It seemed like her breathing always worsened at night or on the weekends, leaving me with the options of an expensive trip to the emergency room or treating her at home using my own judgement. I didn't trust either.

After a few trips to the emergency room and several indecisive times at home, I asked Jaycee's pulmonologist about getting the oxygen saturation monitor so I could see her heart rate and oxygen saturation level. This monitor, which thankfully was paid for by our health insurance, proved its worth time and time again due to her asthma and obstructive sleep apnea.

The monitor gave me two pieces of information that either made me feel better about Jaycee's status or set me off into action. Having experienced the hospital more than a few times, I knew Jaycee's proper heart rate and oxygen saturation level and if she was in some type of distress. It also helped decrease the stress I had taking care of a child who couldn't tell me how she was feeling. The oxygen saturation monitor is a necessary piece of medical equipment that I am thankful Jaycee has in times of illness.

When I didn't think there was anything else to add to our home medical training, then came the vest airway clearance machine. After a few consecutive admissions to the hospital, someone decided Jaycee would benefit from airway clearance due to a poor cough reflex that made her mucus just sit in her lungs. Sometimes she needed to cough but she wouldn't or couldn't. On X-rays, she frequently had atelectasis, which are parts of small collapsed areas in her lungs. Airway clearance could help with these issues.

Respiratory therapy in the hospital started by doing airway clearance or patting her back with cupped hands. It looked simple enough and I was trained on how to continue this procedure at home. I tried these pats during breathing treatments to get Jaycee to cough, often continuing to pat her back in four different spots for a total of eight minutes. I found it was harder than it looked. Perhaps, my arms were just out of shape, but when it needed to be done multiple times a day it could be exhausting.

After tests and several hospital admissions for pneumonia, Jaycee's pulmonologist recommended a vest airway clearance machine. This machine was awesome! Jaycee could wear a vest that buckled in the front with two air hoses attached to either side on the front of the vest; the air hoses attached to a machine that did the airway clearance work with the push of a button. In twenty minutes, the machine could help Jaycee cough and clear her lungs. It sounded like a great idea to me. However, it was difficult to get the machine covered by our insurance.

Even though Jaycee had obstructive sleep apnea, asthma, and multiple respiratory infections requiring hospital admissions, our insurance wouldn't cover the expensive airway clearance machine. Whenever Jaycee was in the hospital, she was able to use one with her breathing treatments, which did seem to help. It was frustrating to be in the hospital with Jaycee over and over for a variety of lung infections and partial lung collapse knowing this machine could possibly prevent some of these admissions if we had one at home.

Finally, during a CT scan of her lungs during one of her hospital admissions, it was discovered Jaycee had a cyst on one of her lungs. It was bad news, another sign that Jaycee's lungs were not healthy. But, I was informed this new diagnosis would allow Jaycee to receive the airway clearance machine with our insurance. It was a diagnosis that brought in mixed emotions, yet, I tried to look on the bright side hoping that the machine would lead to a healthier Jaycee.

When the airway clearance machine took its place in Jaycee's bedroom, it brought more responsibilities with it. On healthy, no symptom days, Jaycee would receive two, 20-minute vest therapy sessions. On days when Jaycee's breathing changed, she received a vest therapy session with every breathing treatment, which was usually every four hours during the day and sometimes throughout the night. This was another adjustment to our daily routine and schedule. It didn't impact me so much as I just had to get her set up on the session and come back twenty minutes later when I needed to take her vest off. But, this required Jaycee to sit still for these sessions, which she was content to do if there was a movie on she could watch. She really handled all the sitting well. The part that was hard for her was getting up earlier in the mornings so she could get her airway clearance session in before leaving for school. Jaycee is not a morning person, so waking her up 20 minutes earlier was like trying to get a bear to wake up out of hibernation. I didn't blame her as I'm not a morning person either. It took some adjusting on her part and patience on mine.

With most every machine added to Jaycee's life, I was accepting if it could potentially help Jaycee stay out of the hospital. I was hopeful if Jaycee caught an innocent cold this new machine would help keep her lungs from developing pneumonia. With this machine, my mentality changed; I didn't think of it as a temporary tool she would eventually outgrow and no longer need. I decided for my own mental well-being that I would just assume she would need airway clearance forever. It was better to accept our new reality instead of being disappointed when a year or two or five went by with Jaycee still needing airway clearance. Five years later, the machine is still used every day, so I was wise to have a better attitude with this piece.

I never imagined my daughter's bedroom would have a BiPAP machine, a nebulizer, an emergency oxygen tank, an oxygen saturation monitor, and a vest airway clearance machine in places where toys, dolls, and books should be. I never pictured a large part of her closet being used to store various nebulizer masks, medications, sensors, cannulas, head gear, and other miscellaneous supplies. But, that's how things have happened and I'm grateful there have been treatments for her.

The training I obtained for this badge set me apart from most other moms; Jaycee proved time and time again to be a unique child. Often, the experiences I had attached to this badge made me feel very isolated as a mother. Being in a rural area, I had not met any mothers who could relate to my experiences with my child. Sometimes, I just needed someone to talk to about these occurrences with Jaycee, but the only people who understood seemed to be people who worked at the hospital.

I took this badge and its knowledge understanding that anything I endured providing care for Jaycee was nothing compared to my sweet girl who endured it all, often without understanding why. But, I did feel like a nurse-in-training at times, as I used all the equipment on my one and only patient, Jaycee.

By: Evana Sandusky

CHAPTER 6:

THE ORGANIZATIONAL SKILLS BADGE

> *Organizational Skills Badge: A mom can earn this badge when she proves she can manage multiple situations, tasks, or appointments when caring for her child. This badge is earned once and is maintained if the mother continues to remember the majority of the important things that need to be done to maintain the child's health, care, or education.*

Organizational Skills Badge Earned: 2006

I have always had a type-A personality. I love schedule books, making lists, and routines. This personality trait may drive my husband crazy at times, but it is helpful for Jaycee's care.

When we took Jaycee home from the hospital after she was born, her health needs were initially overwhelming. I was expecting to take home a healthy baby, settle into motherhood, and return to my job as a school-based speech-language pathologist eight weeks later. The reality was much different and more complex.

When Jaycee was ten days old, we brought her home from the NICU. Jaycee was a "sick" baby that required special care. I think some people assumed because Jaycee was home from the hospital that it was business as usual with my newborn. But it wasn't. Jaycee was battling congestive heart failure, pulmonary hypertension, and low muscle tone.

My organizational skills were pushed to new limits managing Jaycee's care. She was fed every few hours for the first six months of her life. I set alarms to wake myself up at night for feedings because her congestive heart failure made Jaycee sleep more than usual. She never woke up to eat or cried for food **ever** as an infant. Thus, her nutrition depended on me.

With around-the-clock feedings, I was exhausted. The feedings themselves were intense work as her sucking was weak. Without a chance of nursing her, I was lucky to get a few ounces in her with a bottle. There was also no chance of her sleeping through the night, which is the hope of any tired mom. I had to wake her up to make sure she ate enough day and night. Unless my husband took a feeding for me, there was no break and no significant time of rest for Jaycee or myself.

The feedings blurred together, so I kept a notebook to write down when I fed her and how much she drank. I depended on that notebook for months and felt lost without it. The notebook also logged Jaycee's medications. She was on three heart medications given at different times of the day and in different doses—one three times a day, another twice a day, and the last medicine once a day. Sometimes, I would give her a dose but, in my tired state, I'd question whether I really had given it. Like the feedings, the medication times seemed to blur together. The notebook kept me from second guessing myself. I didn't give Jaycee anything without looking at the notebook first and charting it down. If we left the house, the notebook came along too in the diaper bag.

Besides keeping Jaycee's feedings and medicines on schedule, there were numerous appointments to remember. There were regular trips to see the cardiologist and a few trips to the local pediatrician. Early on, a home health nurse came out weekly to monitor Jaycee's health and weight gain. When Jaycee was a few weeks old, she began home therapy through the early intervention program. More people meant more appointments. There were times I wanted to cut things out because I was overwhelmed with everything, but I pushed through knowing all the appointments would not last forever. I always used an appointment book in my pre-mother life, but now Jaycee's medical life depended on it.

The first year of Jaycee's life provided the Organizational Skills Badge over and over. I don't recall ever forgetting an appointment, but I did have a few times when I got the time wrong. Overall, I improved my ability to manage daily tasks and appointments while running a household and trying to bond with my new baby.

Throughout the years, I have continued to use strategies to help me stay organized in Jaycee's care. I no longer need a notebook to track her feedings or daily medications; however, when Jaycee is sick, I still write down the medication times, temperature, and oxygen saturation levels to keep everything scheduled properly and the doctors informed. A schedule book also keeps track of her many specialty appointments, as I refuse to leave anything important for memory.

Another strategy I found helpful early on was doing certain tasks on the same day every week to simplify my duties. Fridays is my equipment cleaning day in which I wash aero chambers for inhalers, nebulizer parts, and BiPAP parts. I check her medications on Friday as well and call in refills as needed. Her medicines are refilled at different times of the month so keeping track of her (presently) nine medications requires attention.

I never imagined I would earn my Organizational Skills Badge by juggling medications, doctors, therapies, and other medical-related duties, but I did. I earned that badge with help from a notebook and scheduler, pen, and sometimes my memory.

By: Evana Sandusky

CHAPTER 7:

THE MISCARRIAGE BADGE

Miscarriage Badge: This badge is given to a mom when she loses a confirmed pregnancy. Unfortunately, this badge can be earned multiple times.

Miscarriage Badge Earned: September 2008

Between the births of my two children, we lost a child. Sometimes, it's easier to pretend my loss didn't occur because it's like opening an old wound. It's not something I talk about often nor is it a subject people bring up in conversation. Never having to speak about it makes it feel less real, I suppose. Miscarriage is a sad and painful part of life that can happen to any woman, me included.

Prior to having children, my husband and I dreamed of having three children. I am not sure why we wanted that number, but for some reason it was stuck in both of our heads.

Jaycee's birth was the first part of our dream fulfillment. Regardless of her diagnoses, we knew we wanted another child. Wanting something and being ready for something is two totally different things. My husband was on board to plan for another child before I was though, and it took some convincing on his part.

To say I was scared to have another child was an understatement. I understood all my risks, especially of having another child with Down syndrome—1%. I wasn't really worried about having another child with Down syndrome; I was worried about any one of the million or more things that could go wrong with a second baby.

My faith in the typical baby experience was shaken, so I was bombarded with thoughts about all sorts of problems. I even worried about having conjoined twins. Ok, that seems strange now that I reflect on it, but it was one of my biggest fears at the time. I was worried one of the baby's limbs would be missing or an organ would not form properly or he or she would have a cleft palate or brain injuries. I was worried about all sorts of things for this future child that I hadn't even started trying to make yet. Before the battle began, my mind had me feeling like I was already losing!

The bottom line was I didn't trust my body—or my genes—anymore. Unlike other women looking to have a baby, I didn't think there were any guarantees with another pregnancy. I had more faith something would be wrong with the next baby and rarely thought I would produce a "typical" child. I would love any child, but I questioned my mental and physical ability to take care of another baby born with high needs.

So, I did what I knew I had to do—I prayed to have another child. I even had people pray with and for me. I confessed to some close prayer warriors that I was nervous about having another child, but they encouraged me. I told Jason about some of my irrational fears and he responded with prayer as well. Eventually, I realized I had to face my fears and go for it. The strong desire to have another child helped ease all those fears away that were almost convincing me not to try.

When my husband and I were finally ready to make Jaycee a big sister, we assumed it would be easy. We got pregnant with Jaycee without really trying so why wouldn't the next try be just as easy? Nothing happened. For eight months, zero babies were made. Jason and I both started to become frustrated but knew it would happen eventually.

I was ecstatic when the pregnancy test finally showed I was pregnant. I was eager for all the things that go with preparing for a baby. As soon as I confirmed the pregnancy with three or possibly four positive tests, I made an appointment with my OB/GYN.

I was scheduled to go to the doctor around the 7th or 8th week into the pregnancy. An early, uncomfortable ultrasound was taken. If you have had an early ultrasound, then you know what I'm talking about. The early stages of a baby was projected onto a screen for us to view and a strong heartbeat was heard. Jaycee, sitting in the room with us, shared in this moment. Since she was not verbal, we knew there was little danger for her to spill the beans to any family members before we were ready to give the news.

Soon after the ultrasound, we decided to tell our families. I am notorious for morning sickness, and I knew I was not going to be able to hide our secret from our parents for too long. Jason and I made up a birth invitation for each of our parents inviting them to come see the new baby on the due date. All our parents were excited and thrilled to have another grandchild coming. I was happy I was able to do a cutesy reveal this time around. It was something I was robbed of the first time, and I was finally going to get that happy moment with smiles and hugs from our family.

News trickled around to other friends and family even though I didn't announce my pregnancy to everyone I bumped into. It wasn't a secret, but it wasn't common knowledge either. I was aware I wasn't out of the danger zone in terms of this pregnancy. I was more concerned about the overall health of the baby and less concerned about a miscarriage.

This pregnancy was different from my previous one. I was not having the extreme morning sickness I had with Jaycee, which I took as a bad sign that my hormones were not high enough. My husband told me to look at it positively and assured me I was fine. If he hadn't, I would have really come completely undone. Known to be a negative thinker, I was hoping Jason was right.

Then I started spotting. I had experienced this with Jaycee, but this too was different. The spotting wasn't severe enough to warrant a trip to the emergency room, but it was enough to cause me anxiety. I was so anxious and sure things weren't going normally. But, I had no proof other than some minor symptoms and a racing mind. Even if I was having a miscarriage, there was nothing I could do. I tried to put on a brave face and continue with life until the next doctor's appointment.

A few days after the spotting started, my husband and I took Jaycee to our town's fall festival celebration. We enjoyed watching Jaycee ride small carnival rides. I even helped her get on and off many of the rides since she was too young to do it on her own. We had a fun night.

When Jason woke up at 4:30 in the morning for work the next day, I was having some cramping. We both felt I had probably overdone it during the festival. He assured me again that I was probably overreacting; I was hopeful he was right. I was 10 weeks along at that point, and I was just ready to be out of the uncertain first trimester.

With both of us not wanting to admit what might be happening, we agreed Jason should go to work. I tried to lay back down and ignore the pains in my stomach. Soon, it was obvious something was not right as I started bleeding heavily. Plus, the cramping felt too much like labor pains.

While my husband was at work, I was home with my 2-year-old having a miscarriage. I woke Jaycee up and got her ready for the day. While she ate breakfast safely in her booster seat, I made multiple trips to the bathroom due to the cramping. I tried to hold myself together for her sake, focusing on Jaycee's needs and maintaining my composure. I called my husband, who was working near the hospital I would eventually be going towards, so we decided to meet at the hospital in a few hours. I called my mom to tell her the bad news.

A short time later, I arrived at my mother's house. I hugged Jaycee goodbye, as my grandmother was there ready to watch her. As my mom and I pulled out of the driveway starting our trek to the hospital about 45 minutes away, I finally allowed all the emotions to come out. I sobbed uncontrollably. I didn't need a doctor to tell me what was happening; it was obvious by that point.

I was so disappointed. It had taken so much courage to try to have another child, and this was a major setback. I didn't know if I had the mental and emotional strength to get through this loss

By: Evana Sandusky

after everything I had already experienced as a parent. This baby was the result of eight months of trying to get pregnant, and I wasn't ready to deal with that stress again. Life didn't seem fair.

By the time mom and I arrived at the emergency room, Jason was there waiting for me. I signed in and took a seat. I wasn't an emergent case, so I sat what seemed like an eternity in the waiting room. I'm not sure how long it actually was but it was more than 30 minutes. When I went to the bathroom, I realized I was losing more and more blood. I asked the woman at the front desk for something to sit on and she swiftly got what I needed and put me in a wheelchair; she also instructed me not to stand up until I was seen by a doctor.

Shortly after that, I was called back to a room. The female nurse seemed to have been through this suspected miscarriage scenario a hundred times before as she ran me through a series of vitals and questions. She was very professional but lacked the compassion that I needed during *my* first experience with a miscarriage.

"Are you on any medications?" she asked as she read through a list of questions.

"No," I responded.

"You aren't on prenatal vitamins?" she questioned, looking over at me.

"Yes, I am," I answered.

"Well, that's a medication," the nurse said as if I was stupid.

That was it—that tiny bit of force in her voice pushed to a place I didn't want to go. I was trying to hold in my emotions at the hospital, even pulling myself together right before I stepped into the emergency room. But at that moment, it was taking all my strength to remain imperturbable.

I choked back the tears until she asked, "Have you been pregnant before?"

I looked at my husband, started crying, and signaled for him to take over the answers from there on out until I got rid of that lump in my throat.

Bloodwork was taken and other routine procedures were performed before I was placed on a monitor since my blood pressure was low. When the nurse finally left the room, I breathed a sigh of relief. I needed a nurse with a little compassion, for which she did not have for me.

Eventually, the doctor came in to do the examination, which was extremely uncomfortable and marginally painful. With a thick accent, he asked me if I knew if I was indeed pregnant. I guess it might be a standard medical question, but I found it odd.

The doctor couldn't say if I had indeed had a miscarriage based on the examination alone, so he ordered an ultrasound for a definite answer. This statement opened the door for hope for a brief period. Maybe it was a language difference or his obscure remark, but my mom, Jason, and I were all under the impression there was a possibility I was still pregnant.

Just after the doctor left, my favorite nurse walked in to check on me. We shared with her our glimmer of hope. She informed us, rather callously, her opinion was I could not be pregnant given the amount of blood I had lost. And just like that, our hope was dissipated once more.

The ultrasound technician was next to arrive, though my family was asked to leave the room for the exam. She claimed having the family outside the room kept people from trying to peek at her screen or ask her a question she was not allowed to answer. I understood, but I was very worried about Jason leaving my side. He and my mom were forced to go back to the waiting room. I was assured when the ultrasound was over they would be notified and escorted back through the locked doors.

The ultrasound was awkward and nerve wrecking. The technician asked me some of the same questions I had answered before with the other professionals, did the exam, and when it was over, she left. I was alone for what seemed like ages; all I wanted was my family with me. My thoughts were swirling about and it felt like everyone had forgotten I was in the room. Not one nurse or medical staff member even came in to check on me and I was left to deal with the anxiety of our loss alone.

I was about to have a panic attack in that small, enclosed room. Plus, I was too weak to get out of the bed. Little did I know, Jason was worried, too. He knew how long ultrasounds should take and it was taking much too long. He asked the receptionist if he could be escorted back to see me but was told someone needed to verify I could receive visitors. I was not sure who was responsible for reporting the information, but it was not done. Finally, after about an hour, a nurse came in the room asking the whereabouts of my family. *Good question!* Within minutes, they were allowed back.

I was given medication to stop my bleeding after it was confirmed I had miscarried. There was no longer a baby, no longer a pregnancy.

I was monitored a little while longer since my blood pressure was still low but then released to go home with strict orders for bed rest until I saw my physician in a few days. I was somewhat surprised that during the entire time in the hospital no one had any regard for my mental and emotional well-being. It was purely the medical aspect and the coping was left to my own abilities.

When we reached my house, I was physically and mentally exhausted, not to mention still cramping and very much in the middle of my miscarriage. I immediately grabbed the television remote and rested on the couch. On the television was a rerun of a sitcom I thought would take my mind off of things. Instead, I was dumbfounded and livid when the character in the comedy show had a miscarriage. The episode was all about her loss and moving on. *What are the chances?* I quickly changed the channel but took it as a sign that I was not alone in this experience.

Over the next few days, I tried to take it easy. My family helped with Jaycee's care. I spent my free time trying to keep from crying. It was a difficult job! I sent a few text messages and emails to close friends and family to tell them what happened, figuring the word would spread around. For the most part it worked though I had a few awkward moments in the weeks to come when asked about my pregnancy.

At my OB/GYN appointment a few days later, another ultrasound was taken showing the same results, however, at least no further procedures were needed, for which I was thankful. Another unexpected event that day was the personal talk with my OB/GYN. I shared with him how my first child had Down syndrome and now this pregnancy was a miscarriage. My biggest concern was if there was something wrong with me.

"No, you just have really bad luck. There's no reason why the next pregnancy won't be completely normal," he assured me.

That was exactly what I needed to hear. He encouraged me to try again and was upbeat about future pregnancies. His nurse informed me if I wanted to try again to wait two cycles before doing so, as it should be easier to conceive if we start trying quickly after this loss—another relief. I will never forget the compassionate doctor and nurse who reinvigorated my desire to conceive again.

The physical healing after that loss lasted a few weeks. My stomach, which had swollen during the miscarriage, went down. I regained my energy and returned to work after having a week or so off. The emotional healing, on the other hand, took much longer. Every time I heard of a pregnancy, saw a pregnant woman, or saw a sweet baby, I just wanted to cry. I found myself hopelessly jealous of people who could make healthy babies. I had tried twice to have a healthy baby and neither time went according to plan. *Why was it so hard for me?*

Those who had related stories of their own miscarriages were an inspiration to me as well. I was surprised how many people had experienced this loss and their stories normalized it for me. A friend lent me a book on miscarriage; reading the common emotions and thoughts after a loss helped me understand my own feelings.

I wanted to do something to remember this child whose life only existed inside of me briefly. For a few short weeks, this baby provoked dreams for the future in my head. I tried not to get too attached, but it happened naturally, as soon as the pregnancy test read positive. For people to insinuate the pregnancy was forgettable was impossible for me. I felt robbed not knowing the baby's gender in order to name him or her. In fact, it seemed the grayish blob ultrasound picture taken earlier in my pregnancy was the only remaining evidence of this baby.

Rather than framing that ultrasound picture or putting it somewhere to be seen often, I decided to remember this baby with an ornament for our Christmas tree. I found one of an angel with a small child in front of it. It seemed like the perfect way to memorialize our baby. Every Christmas when I place this ornament on our tree, I take a moment to remember the loss and to be thankful for the children I do have.

I have moved on from that dark time in my life as a mother. This badge was never one I wanted nor expected yet once given, it could never be undone nor forgotten. I struggled emotionally for a bit after receiving this badge. The sadness endured for quite some time, along with a wide range of other emotions. Time did heal the emotional wounds attached to the badge. It was hard to live through, but the raw emotions are no longer there.

By: Evana Sandusky

Fortunately, my next pregnancy with Elijah went as planned, and I had a healthy baby to hold. The pain and loss from the miscarriage healed significantly when I held Elijah. He was an answer to our prayers in so many ways. My heart feels heavy for other moms who experienced a miscarriage and did not have baby later to console them. For all of the mothers who have more than one of these badges, my deepest condolences. Remember, your loss is real and your pain is valid, but you will endure and rise up once more. Hopefully, we will all meet our unborn babies in Heaven one day.

CHAPTER 8:

THE COURAGE BADGE

> *Courage Badge: This badge is earned when a mom displays an incredible amount of strength to carry on through a difficult parenting experience with positivity. Sometimes, a mom is aware she is displaying great courage; other times, she realizes she had courage after the fact. A mom can only receive one badge, though it can be lost and re-earned multiple times.*

Courage Badge Earned: 2006

After Jaycee was born, the countdown to her open-heart surgery began. It was the first time in my life that I truly comprehended stress. Before this, I would shake my head about news stories reporting on people struggling with stress. I had no idea, and I couldn't relate. What circumstance could be so stressful that it could affect your own health? I was about to find out as a 26-year-old mother.

The three months between delivering Jaycee and waiting for her heart surgery were both joyous and dreadful. I was weighed down with so many emotions while being so in love with my daughter. Her soft skin, her sweet baby noises, and her small features all made her irresistible. I loved dressing her up in all her pretty, new clothes and taking in motherhood for the first time. But, the medications for her congestive heart failure were a daily reminder that those things could all end if her heart surgery was not successful.

My husband and I tried to remain positive, prayed for a good outcome, and encouraged others to do the same. I earned my Courage Badge during that trying time of uncertainty. For three months, fear, stress, and worry tried to make appearances into my life and mind. I fought hard against those, trying not to be negative. I spent hours each week praying for Jaycee, speaking scriptures from the Bible, and making good confessions. I felt led to go on a 7-day fast for Jaycee. Normally, fasting (going without food) was difficult for me, but that time was different. I was motivated to seek God on behalf of my daughter and pray for her to have a long and healthy life. Looking back, I think that fast had less to do with Jaycee and more about God teaching me things about myself.

I learned that being courageous doesn't mean doubts are nonexistent. They were still there, I just had to fight them off. I felt I was doing well in that fight, most of the time.

I ricocheted between praying faithful prayers and crying with worry. I tried to stay optimistic about the situation but then caught myself studying Jaycee's breathing for signs of worsening congestive heart failure. The thought of her dying during surgery or her heart failure worsening before surgery plagued me every day. I was apprehensive her pulmonary hypertension was doing irreversible damage or that she would need a pacemaker after surgery, which would forever change her life. I was constantly in a battle of positivity versus reality. The reality was she was a sick baby, but I desperately wanted her to be okay.

My motherly instinct told me everything would be fine. Somehow, I knew Jaycee would live a long life. I had to stay in the fight so my daughter could fight. Giving up and totally succumbing to the concern, fear, and stress would have meant the Courage Badge wouldn't be mine. I fought, and I was winning, even if I didn't always feel like it.

By: Evana Sandusky

When Jaycee made it through her heart surgery, I was relieved, which allowed all the uncertainty about her life to vanish. I looked forward to her future and knew life would get easier. I never imagined motherhood would bring me so many hard-earned badges.

After I received my Courage Badge for the first time as a mother, there was opportunity after opportunity for me to keep the badge. Each health scare or diagnosis that came up was an occasion for me to hold on tight to my badge or to lose it. You can imagine after reading through the previous chapters in this book how difficult it was to stay positive about Jaycee's health and future. There were many days I wanted to stay in bed, pretend like I didn't have any problems, and emotionally detach from everything. But, I didn't; I couldn't. Jaycee needed me to be strong. For the most part, I held on to my Courage Badge with only small moments of anguish and negativity.

There were times when I absolutely lost my bravery. Sometimes, I was not even aware it was gone. I kept finding myself in situations with Jaycee that slowly caused me to become more pessimistic and anxious. I could not even pray with the intensity I had before. I always wanted Jaycee to be healthy and live, but every illness and complication thrown her way made it more arduous to believe it was going to happen. I had strong doubts of seeing her live long enough to hit certain moments in time that all parents dream about. When the dreams seemed more like wishes that might not come true, my courage faded away little by little until being positive was not possible.

Without my Courage Badge, life was harder. In 2011, when Jaycee was diagnosed with Wolff-Parkinson-White (WPW) syndrome, the months between the diagnosis and the heart ablations were excruciating. If the time before her first open heart surgery was unbearable, this was a million times worse. The idea an electrical pathway in her heart could trigger at any moment for no reason or cause sudden death snapped my resolve. I understood the possibility of it happening was low, but it was still a possibility.

Any silence during the day was immediately filled with the plaguing thought, "Is Jaycee ok right now in this moment?" With all the things I had been through with Jaycee, I had never felt the stress spill over into all areas of my life. But this was different; the stress was unrelenting, finding its way into my head space almost every waking moment.

I didn't seek out too many people to pray about Jaycee this time. I could barely talk about the situation without breaking down. People thought I was strong; I guess I believed them but even strong people need help and encouragement from others at times. Looking back, I should have sought people out to discuss my qualms; perhaps that would have minimized the power those worrisome thoughts had in my life. Instead, I pretended like things were ok—but they were far from it.

Something was different yet I couldn't understand what it was until I looked at my sash. My Courage Badge was missing! *At what point did my courage leave me?* I couldn't pinpoint the exact time. I just knew that in my current state negative, anxious, and fearful thoughts were abundant, and my courage was nowhere to be found. *Where was that part of me that was able to be positive in hard situations? Where was the dauntless person whose faith knew Jaycee would live through her heart surgery?* That courage seemed long gone, almost as if it never belonged to me. I felt like a different person for most of 2011.

Really, I was not myself. She was diagnosed with WPW in January and her first ablation was in May. I was very relieved when that ablation was over, so life could return to normal. I almost instantly felt my courage return. With the threat of death gone, I could appreciate how we all survived this unfortunate "test." I was hopeful about our future as a family as the battles were ending in our favor. *Why did I ever doubt and lose courage?*

Then in June, the news came that her WPW returned on the EKG. Just like that my courage was gone again. *Here we go!* Same old worries, same old fears, same old struggles, and same poor response by me! I was worn out in every way. I felt so ecstatic when the WPW was gone and now the exact opposite emotion was on me. Maybe I should have worked harder to control my negative thoughts. After all, Jaycee had made it that long without another WPW trigger. But, my mind seemed to revert back, and I just allowed it to run in that opposite direction.

After Jaycee's second successful ablation a few months later, my courage came back for good. It was not instant, as I became a more guarded person. For a time, I was leery about being too positive and setting myself up to be smacked right back down again by another crisis. The roller coaster of emotions drained me as I was unprepared for all the health battles my child faced. But then again, who would be? I wanted to be a normal parent with normal problems, not constantly in scary health crises in which my daughter's life was always questionable.

I slowly began to discover and accept our normal. Jaycee's life was a series of diagnoses, hospital admissions, surgeries, medications, and apparatuses. It didn't define her life, but it was a regular part of it. When I realized that fact, my bitterness and out-of-control emotions and thinking faded. I knew it would happen, and eventually our life would go back to its normal. That mentality helped my courage to abide.

Every situation I have been in with Jaycee just prepares me for another challenge in the future. I did come out stronger after each challenge; I seldom recognized it at the time though. Although, when Jaycee was at her sickest, I knew exactly where my courage was because my daughter needed it.

When Jaycee was near death in the ICU in 2013, my Courage Badge remained strongly attached to my sash. Of course, I had occasional moments of breakdown, but I endured them with strength and determination. I guess when you are told your child may not live, the only thing you have left is your hope that somehow things will turn out fine. That is what I decided to do in that moment—believe she would live.

As she lay in that hospital bed sedated and breathing on a ventilator, I projected my courage and strength onto my daughter. Perhaps the trial with WPW and my negativity taught me that courage was the only and best way to make it through a difficult situation. I rose to the occasion once again.

I prayed for Jaycee. I read scriptures over her. I spoke positive affirmations about her life to her. I did similar things that earned me the Courage Badge in the first place. When a scary event happened during that four-week hospital stay, I took a breath, cried if necessary, and then moved forward, checking to make sure my Courage Badge was still on my sash.

I have walked through situations with Jaycee with strength and weakness—and we survived. I can tell you trying to be courageous by squashing negative thoughts is the only way to fight those battles. A Courage Badge does not mean that fear, stress, and pessimism isn't present. It simply means these emotions are not winning. I strive to let courage win and I encourage you to as well.

By: Evana Sandusky

CHAPTER 9:

THE SECOND LANGUAGE BADGE

Second Language Badge: When a mom must learn a second language to parent her child, this badge is earned. This is not a badge earned for an elective second language, but is reserved for moms who must learn their own language for essential communication with their child.

Second Language Badge Earned: 2008

Prior to having Jaycee, I knew some sign language since I used it from time to time in my job as a pediatric speech-language pathologist. I never dreamed I would become dependent on it to communicate with my child one day.

As a baby, Jaycee rarely babbled. I remember being excited when she jabbered "dada" for the first time, but nothing much came after that. Eventually even that stopped. As a toddler, she was mostly quiet with an occasional babble or word as her language was delayed due to her Down syndrome.

When Jaycee was around 18-months old, sign language was introduced to her because it is often a successful strategy for children with Down syndrome. I signed to her and nothing happened for what seemed like a long time, but in retrospect, it was probably only a month or two. In addition to signing to her, I helped her form the signs by using a hand-over-hand method and watched signing DVDs together. The first time she signed "more" was magical.

She continued learning a sign here and there. I became disappointed and impatient, most likely because if she couldn't speak, her ability to learn and use sign language would give me some insight into her intellect and memory. To me, her lack of speech and signs was troublesome. I continued trying to teach speech or signs while she received help by another trained speech-language pathologist, too.

One day, I had a breakthrough with her. Some of Jaycee's signing DVDs came with an accompanying CD of the music. We had watched the movies over and over, so I wanted to switch things up. When the theme song came through the speakers Jaycee waddled to the television screen confused. She recognized the music but didn't understand why the screen was black. It upset her because she wanted to see her show. In a short time, though, she had figured out the source of the sound came from the speaker and she was happy. As one familiar song after another played, Jaycee started doing something I never expected—signing many new signs I never knew she had retained!

I had been so frustrated that my child wasn't learning signs at a rate I expected when the reality was she was retaining them after all! Once the visual of the television screen was taken away, she was signing along to those songs she knew so well. Plus, I couldn't believe how many signs she knew. I started to write them down to remember which ones to use with her later. That day changed my perspective on Jaycee and her ability to learn and use sign language. It also reminded me that if something doesn't appear to be working, try presenting it in a slightly different way. After I realized what she knew, I incorporated the signs into her everyday life.

Soon, I was ordering more and more signing DVDs to keep her vocabulary growing. I eventually taught her the colors and alphabet in sign, which she caught on to quickly. Because she showed an interest in animals, we used flashcards to provide her a picture of the animal we were naming by sign. By the time Jaycee was three years old, she could only say a couple of words but was signing at least 200 words. It was a challenge for me to keep learning new signs but seeing Jaycee use them and learn new words was motivating and exciting.

I loved seeing her sign "horse" as we passed horses standing in a field as we drove down the highway. We laughed as she signed "tigers scared" at random times reminding us that she feared tigers. We aren't sure where this fear of tigers came from, but it was a sign phrase she used for years and years. Watching her sign the foods on her plate like "chicken, corn, potatoes" followed by a verbal "mmm" was amazing and made our lives as parents feel a little more "normal." Sign language allowed Jaycee's thoughts and personality to come through and express herself. Earning my Second Language Badge is exciting when it means you finally have a way to communicate with your child.

Second Language Badge Earned: 2011

There came a point when sign language became inefficient. Jaycee was thriving with it, but there were some problems since hardly anyone knows sign language, limiting her communication partners. Even if a person did know sign language, many of Jaycee's signs were only approximations due to her fine motor limitations. Therefore, people did not recognize Jaycee's version of the sign. Plus, I was completely out of signs to teach her and couldn't keep up with her "demand" for new words. She seemed to remember the new signs better than I did!

Using sign language daily also showed me more issues with that method. Communication in the dark, such as movie theaters, was near impossible. Jaycee liked to communicate about things she saw as we drove in a vehicle also, which became a problem when I was driving as she wanted me to look at her signs when it wasn't safe for me to do so.

Once when driving Jaycee to St. Louis for a doctor's appointment she kept repeating "momma" as we drove over a tall bridge. I looked back briefly to see her sign "boat water." I shook my head "yes" at her and then it quickly shifted to a big "NO," as I turned my eyes forward again to see traffic suddenly stopped in front of me. Yes, there is a time and a place for sign language—traffic is not one of them!

When she was five, it was clear Jaycee wasn't going to develop verbal speech any time soon as she was quite delayed, even for Down syndrome. Sign language was initially started as a temporary method of communication while her verbal speech developed. It had become evident Jaycee needed a new system to allow better communication with people. I was debating on what to do next when I stumbled onto my next option.

Sometimes things in life just work out. As I was deciding how to help Jaycee next, I attended a work-related training on hearing loss and cochlear implants being conducted by a team of people from St. Louis Children's Hospital. One of them was a very knowledgeable speech-language pathologist (SLP) who really impressed me. I felt like I was attending this training to meet this person to get some guidance for my own daughter. I patiently waited around after the training to speak to her for a few minutes. She seemed genuinely interested in trying to get Jaycee some help but said her co-worker was better suited to handle our case, as she had more experience with children with Down syndrome.

After exchanging a few emails with this recommended SLP, I made an appointment for an evaluation at the hospital. In one email she asked me if I had ever considered a speech generating communication device. *Huh?* I was floored but I should not have been. I was hoping this SLP would have some magical trick that would increase Jaycee's verbal speech since I had convinced myself there wasn't something in my professional background to help Jaycee speak. Surely, I believed my child would speak and her lack of speech would not be forever. Getting a communication device seemed to suggest that maybe that would be the case.

So, I did what any professional woman would do—researched, read, and thought. I didn't email the SLP back quickly regarding the communication device as I needed to process the question and decide what it would mean for Jaycee and for myself. All in all, I had to face the truth that this would most likely benefit all of us. It would be a change, but I was open to it. I was familiar with the benefits of devices from my education and had to give it serious consideration. I looked

By: Evana Sandusky

forward to Jaycee's language evaluation and the professional's thoughts on what we should do next.

The SLP set Jaycee's language on a new course. Jaycee was diagnosed with Childhood Apraxia of Speech, which occurs in about 10-15% of children with Down syndrome. The diagnosis didn't surprise me as I had suspected this for some time myself, but she did caution me that Jaycee would have to work extremely hard to pick up any verbal speech as her apraxia was severe. She wisely explained Jaycee's future couldn't be predicted but the chances of her one day speaking clearly and in full sentences was slim. I was relieved to have someone be so honest and forthcoming about expectations for Jaycee.

She suggested we give a speech generating communication device a chance. Being a SLP myself, I understood and agreed with her point of view, but I wanted **MY** daughter to talk. The magical fix I was searching for just didn't exist; deep down, I knew it.

We soon found ourselves with a one-month borrowed device that we referred to as Jaycee's "talker." As we waited for the insurance to decide on funding her own device, the loaner device allowed us to see if we really wanted it before all the paperwork went through.

Jaycee's loaner talker had a screen with icons representing categories of words and phrases. Pictures of family members, favorite foods, or television shows were added to help customize it. Words Jaycee didn't have signs for became important to me during this trial process. With the push of a button, Jaycee had access to many words the device would speak for her.

Using this device was like learning a second language. I had to understand the icons, memorize word locations, and spend time programming the device to make it personal for Jaycee. It was important for me to know how to use the device because I had to model words and phrases for Jaycee.

During the month-long trial, it became apparent the talker was going to enhance Jaycee's ability to communicate with others and opened a whole new set of words for her. For instance, she previously signed "cousin" to represent any one of her cousins. Now, by adding a photo and the name of each cousin to the device, she could talk about each cousin individually. Beyond that, we programmed a prayer into her device that allowed her to now take part in our faith. Jaycee frequently said "pizza" on her talker, which was when I discovered pizza, and not chicken nuggets, was her favorite food. For whatever reason, Jaycee was requesting things for the first time; this clued us into her favorite color (green) and people she favored more because she was pushing those buttons on her talker often. She never really did this with sign language, and I'm not sure why the talker made the difference, but it advanced her communication skills almost immediately.

When the trial was over, it was clear to everyone in the family that Jaycee *needed* this device. Prior to the trial, some family members had their doubts and worried Jaycee's verbal speech would stop if we started using it. There were other concerns too, but no one could deny how well Jaycee communicated with the device. That's what all of us wanted!

When her very own device arrived, Jaycee began using it immediately, proving it was a good decision. However, sign language still had a place in our life since a device isn't practical in every situation. For instance, communication while swimming or bathing cannot be on an electronic device. Sign language was Jaycee's first language, so it is instinctive for her to use it, even now.

With that device purchase came another opportunity to earn a Second (or is it third now) Language Badge. I never thought I would have to learn how to use one of these for my own child, but her improvement in communication was worth all the research and work.

At 12 years old, Jaycee is encouraged to use a total communication approach at home, which means she uses signs, verbal speech, gestures, and her talker. Her verbal speech began making the biggest strides around age 10, and she's saying new words regularly. Her talker is used less and less as her verbal speech improves, but it is still needed in her life, just like sign language.

All those years ago I thought I wanted my daughter to speak, and I did, but I really wanted to communicate with her; this badge helped me do just that.

CHAPTER 10:

THE FORGIVENESS BADGE

> *Forgiveness Badge: A mom earns this badge when she forgives someone who has hurt her in respect to her role as a mother. A Forgiveness Badge is awarded one time when a mom decides to forgive someone. However, if she chooses to hold a grudge against someone, then she must re-earn her badge by practicing forgiveness.*

Forgiveness Badge Initially Earned: 2006

Forgiveness seems to be something that I do more frequently as Jaycee's mother versus Elijah's mother. There are far more opportunities for offensive comments, interactions, and situations with people than with Elijah because there are many more people involved in Jaycee's care. There have been numerous doctors, nurses, special education teachers, teacher's aides, and therapists who have been around Jaycee and me, which means infinite situations for these people to discuss my child, my parenting, and my family life overall. I could find off-putting, hurtful, insulting, or irrational comments or statements made during any one of the numerous encounters. People can say the wrong thing even if they mean well. It's bound to happen to anyone, but when your child has a team of specialists around her I found it occurred more often than not.

Besides just the sheer number of people who may share some hurtful words regarding my daughter, the fact that Jaycee has a developmental disability opens her and me up to other unwanted ideas. She is subject to society's thoughts, assumptions, and beliefs about people with disabilities. Many people are uneducated about disabilities or Jaycee's health problems, but that has not stopped them from having opinions. Their fearlessness and often cruel views about those with developmental disabilities are always shared online as well. I have been taken back by some things strangers, acquaintances, and doctors have said over the years.

From the moment Jaycee was diagnosed, I had opportunities to exercise forgiveness. The doctor's information about Jaycee having Down syndrome told me, among other things, that Jaycee wouldn't look like me, which affected me more than I care to admit. I believed this man who gave me a half-truth. Sure, she had features of Down syndrome, but my genetics were there, too. When I finally came to realize Jaycee did look like me, I found myself very angry at the man who gave me such poor information. Years later, I realized just how much his words hurt me, and that I was holding a large grudge against him. I had to pray about it and release those hurts. I prayed for that doctor to have the wisdom to better interact with parents in the future. He is just one example of a person in the medical field who needed my forgiveness, even though he never knew it.

There have been many well-meaning Christian people whom I had to forgive. There were a few people who suggested Jaycee was demon-possessed because of her Down syndrome; they saw Down syndrome as something that needed healing and not something to be embraced. Some insisted my husband or I must have sinned to bring these diagnoses into her life. Again, Down syndrome was looked at negatively, as punishment, and not an opportunity to care for someone other than myself. Both attitudes in the church were all extremely difficult to hear. I had to get

By: Evana Sandusky

past my hurt feelings and look at their intentions. People wanted Jaycee to be whole, which was good, but they approached us in an insensitive way and had a worldview about disability that differed from mine.

The prayers that my fellow Christians prayed over Jaycee to be healed of her Down syndrome repeatedly became a source of contention for me in church. *Did she have to be "normal" to be accepted in my faith?* Countless people spoke to me about God and his mysterious ways left me feeling beat down and more confused. I felt there were less and less people I could engage in conversation with that first year of Jaycee's life for fear of them saying something to offend me. I had to forgive these people and learn to socialize again.

Outside the church, there was even more forgiveness needed. Comments regarding Jaycee's lack of progress somehow being my fault became imprinted into my mind. Certain people who said things like, "Jaycee doesn't walk because she has first child syndrome," left me in a puddle of tears. It didn't matter to them that Jaycee wasn't expected to walk until closer to age two with her Down syndrome diagnosis, as that, too, was somehow my fault.

Other people over the years suggested Jaycee's lack of verbal speech was somehow due to my husband and I not teaching her to speak or modeling it for her; these small comments made Jason and I feel like people perceived us as part of Jaycee's problem. They couldn't comprehend that her delays were the result of a combination of factors they didn't even inquire about nor witnessed any of the therapy and techniques we tried with Jaycee on our own and with professionals in sessions. Yes, I had to forgive these people who made me feel like a bad parent and hurt my feelings.

Then there were people who seemed to be nosey about our situation with Jaycee. One time, we went out to McDonald's for breakfast to celebrate my birthday. I held little 3-month-old Jaycee in my arms taking in the moment and trying to forget about her heart surgery in less than a week. Someone I recognized but don't know well sat across the restaurant and asked, "When's her heart surgery?"

"Next week," I answered. That was the conversation. They had no follow-up comments or words of support. They didn't even have the decency to walk over and talk to me privately about it. This may seem petty to most people, but this interaction bothered me for months. I felt she was just being meddlesome and didn't consider I might not want to shout out a response about my baby's heart surgery in McDonald's. Situations like that caused me to be leery of public appearances during stressful moments in Jaycee's life. Yet, this woman also deserved my forgiveness, even though she didn't even know she needed it.

I have had to forgive complete strangers over the years, like the people who stared at my child in public and made us feel like a spectacle. Eventually, I stopped letting it bother me and forgave those who unknowingly offended me. When Jaycee was a baby, strangers often approached me and asked if she had Down syndrome as they usually had a relative with Down syndrome and wanted to share a quick exchange. I often found these encounters annoying as I just wanted to be out in public like anyone else and not focus on my child's extra chromosome. One stranger in the grocery store remarked on Jaycee's red skin tone and asked if she had a rash. I'm not sure if that person was a germaphobe or a doctor, but either way, I thought the comment was strange. For a time, I dreaded going in out in public, but I eventually reached a place where I could allow people to be curious and walk in forgiveness.

I have had to forgive children for the way they have treated Jaycee. When I see children playing a game I have termed "Run from Jaycee." It upsets me knowing Jaycee thinks she's involved in a fun game of chase when really the object is for everyone to run away from her. Even if Jaycee isn't hurt from the child's game because she doesn't understand their cruelty, I am. When children push Jaycee out of their area and don't include her, it irks me. When children roll their eyes when Jaycee follows them around, I want to surround Jaycee in a big hug as I plot long reprimands in my head of what I would like to say to those children.

In the end, I realize I am expecting too much from other children. A mom never wants to see her child excluded but it will probably happen with any child regardless if he or she has special needs. I must remind myself as a child I was never one to befriend children with special needs. *How can I be mad at a child who doesn't understand everything about Jaycee?* There are many adults, often parents themselves, who don't know how to interact with her. Therefore, I have forgiven children multiple times for things they did or said to my daughter.

Over the years, I have had to forgive people who didn't offer support the way I envisioned it. Initially, we had a ton of backing from family and friends after Jaycee was born. There were numerous cards, monetary and food donations, and people visiting—it was wonderful and helpful. As time went on, we experienced less and less support during her health crises. I expected certain family members or friends to show up at the hospital or, at the very least, contact us by phone when an emergency arose only to be let down. With texting available, there was little excuse for not reaching out. When people didn't make any efforts, I assumed they didn't care. I became mad and disappointed with people time and time again when they didn't perform to my expectations. People, who told me how much Jaycee meant to them and how they loved her, were not even contacting us during times of serious illness. Actions speak louder than words to me. *Where was everyone when we needed them? Didn't people care? Didn't they know how serious her problems were?*

I thought if the situation was reversed how they would love to have support from others. Truthfully, many of my relationships changed because of our experiences with Jaycee. Some people stepped up and came on the scene to provide encouragement while others did not. I didn't want things from people, but I did want their love, or to hear they were praying for us, or just to know they cared. But I slowly learned to focus on the people who *did* step up for us instead of focusing on those who were absent. People will let you down. I'm sure I have not lived up to someone's expectations either. Sometimes, I am unsure of what to say to someone or how to approach them when they are dealing with a crisis so, I stay away thinking it would be best for both of us. That's not the right approach, but one I have erroneously taken time and time again. With that in mind, I had to forgive certain friends, church members, and family members; they have their own lives and are doing their best. I don't always respond well to people, so I need to extend grace to others that I need for myself.

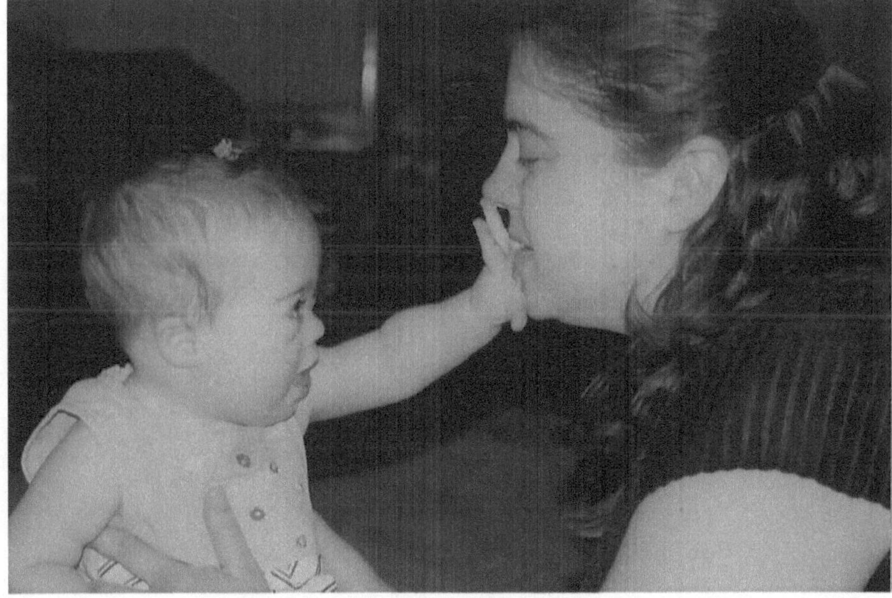

Jaycee and Mommy in 2006

By: Evana Sandusky

Walking in forgiveness is so important. As Jaycee's mother, I have a full plate of responsibilities. I can't let petty grudges, little comments, actions, or inactions take away my joy. No one is perfect, especially not me. Everyone deserves forgiveness.

Truth be told, it was difficult for me to forgive people when they hurt me in the beginning. I didn't necessarily want to hold a grudge, but it's hard to let go of that hurt. Letting go seems as if I'm saying my hurt wasn't valid. Whether it's valid or not, forgiveness is necessary to live a happier life.

Basically, earning the Forgiveness Badge is arduous. Maintaining it is even more difficult. While everyone deserves forgiveness, not everyone deserves my time. If there is someone who consistently upsets me and doesn't treat Jaycee well, then I choose not to spend my time with that person, if possible. If I don't connect with a doctor, I can find another one. I try to use common sense in protecting Jaycee and myself nowadays.

I try to remember that everyone makes mistakes and deserves a second chance. I want to keep my Forgiveness Badge and keep peace in my life.

CHAPTER 11:

THE FAITH BADGE

> *Faith Badge: This badge is earned when a mother clings to her religious beliefs through child-related trials that have the potential to destroy it. Only one badge is awarded, though it can be lost and re-earned if needed.*

Faith Badge Initially Earned: 2006

I grew up in a Christian family and knew Jesus as my personal savior for many years. When I was pregnant with Jaycee, I was in my second year as a youth leader at our church, teaching on Wednesday evenings and helping to plan different youth functions. At that time, I was very involved in church life and, more importantly, had an extremely close relationship with God.

Looking back, I see the time before Jaycee was born was crucial to my faith, as God was preparing me for what was going to happen. Before getting pregnant, I had been fasting monthly, as I felt, at the time, it was something I should do. I had a strong prayer life and was faithful in my Bible reading as well. I loved God and was quick to encourage and pray for those going through difficult circumstances. I knew God was real and considered myself a positive and faithful person. Little did I know, it was all preparation for the obstacles ahead. God knew my strength, emotions, and faith would be challenged, so laying the groundwork before the trial was crucial.

When Jaycee was born and the diagnoses were given, I can't fully explain how I felt. Almost every emotion and thought possible was going on inside of me at that time. I was happy to be a mother but also quickly went into a deep depression from the shock of the circumstances I found myself in. I worried about my marriage holding up due to the perceived strain of raising a child with developmental and medical needs. The apprehension of Jaycee dying and, in the same moment, how I would care for her as she got older were concerns as well. I wondered how I was going to work and care for this medically-fragile baby. There were so many mindsets and qualms but my faith was crucial to me staying sane.

The biggest question I had for God after Jaycee was born was, "Why didn't I know when I was pregnant?"

I really didn't ask "Why did this happen to me?" Well, I probably did ask that but really, I was hurt the God I prayed to daily did not give me any indication and/or warning as to the problems that were about to unfold when Jaycee was born. I felt blind sighted by the diagnoses and the life altering news for me and my family.

Why wasn't something caught on the ultrasound? Why didn't I realize that the little movement I felt while I carried Jaycee wasn't normal? Why didn't the doctor ask me more questions?

The passage of time allows a fresh perspective on things. Now, I understand there never would have been a "good" time to find out about Jaycee's health issues. If I had known before I delivered Jaycee, I could have prepared myself by reading up on her health conditions and by delivering her at a hospital that was prepared to care for a baby like her. But, that was about it. I would have taken the news hard no matter when I received it.

Frankly, I'm glad I didn't know until she was born. I have happy memories of baby showers and people being so excited for me. I know those interactions would have had a different feeling if everyone had known Jaycee wasn't going to be the picture of health. I also confess that I would have been emotionally a wreck had I known while I was pregnant. The news wouldn't have been easy for me to handle as I was trying to work at my school job and prepare at home for the baby.

By: Evana Sandusky

Now, I know it was a good plan for me not to have any warning. But after Jaycee was born, it was a hard thing to accept. I had prayed for a healthy child during my pregnancy. My prayers felt unanswered when Jaycee was diagnosed. My faithful prayers all those months felt moot. My faith was shaken, and I didn't quite know how to view Jaycee's diagnosis because my emotions and shock overtook everything in the beginning. I had arrived in a place where bad things happen in life and felt God was powerless in the situation. Yet, I never stopped asking God what He thought about Jaycee's diagnoses and how I needed to view them.

With questions and concerns looming in my mind, the biggest battle I faced beyond her diagnoses was Jaycee's first open heart surgery when she was three months old. At that time, I was feeding Jaycee around-the-clock, giving her medications several times a day, dealing with medical appointments and home health visits, feeling utterly exhausted, and having post-partum hormones. I was trying to figure out who I was and how to be a new mom while dealing with all those stressors.

Even though I had many questions, I pressed on to earn my Faith Badge. I prayed for Jaycee to be protected and healthy, and I prayed she would be healed and not have to go through the surgery. I felt it was the right way to pray at the time, so that's how I prayed.

I felt led to go on a fast for Jaycee before her surgery. Amidst the fears I had, I wanted to focus my life on interceding for Jaycee's life. I spent a week not eating any food and limited myself on what liquids I drank. Before this, the longest I had ever fasted was three days, and I found those fasts extremely hard. This was much longer, but I found this time was easier as it allowed me to focus my thoughts onto Jaycee. The fast happened to fall during Mother's Day so instead of eating with my family to celebrate my first Mother's Day, it was a simple time of reflection and prayer. By the end of the fast, I felt ready to take on Jaycee's health issues knowing God was there beside us.

After the fast ended, I continued to read scriptures and placed them all over the house. I immersed myself in my faith while still having a wide range of emotions that tried to pull me in a different direction spiritually.

When Jaycee went in for her heart surgery, I was at peace. I had prayed all I could pray, and it wasn't in my hands anymore. Jaycee wasn't supernaturally healed, but I felt ok. I didn't understand everything that had happened, but I was at peace during her 4-hour surgery.

After Jaycee's heart surgery, I had unrealistic expectations. I thought once her surgery was completed, she would change drastically, and things would get easier. I thought she would drink more and faster. But, the feeding schedule was still as intense, as she continued to be a poor feeder. She was on oxygen for a few months post-surgery and still need many doctor's appointments. I was still exhausted mentally and physically, something I wasn't expecting post-surgery. When your body and mind are pushed to their limit, something is bound to happen. I found myself in utter depression.

For me, the battle with depression was as if I was lost and helpless in the middle of an ocean. I pictured myself treading water in an endless sea constantly trying to stay afloat. There was no land or rescue ship anywhere in sight and my treading left me worn out. At times, I got temporary relief from an object that I found floating in the waters. But mysteriously that object always got away from me and I was once again treading water with no hope of a way out in sight. I knew I needed to keep afloat to stay alive, but I felt powerless to change the situation. My body was exhausted from the daily struggles, and I wanted nothing more than to be at peace.

I became a different person due to depression. When I was alone, I cried. In the shower or on a car ride, I would cry. You must understand that prior to this, I was a person who rarely ever cried. My family is not known as the touchy, feely, emotional type. I was that way, too.

Sometimes, Jason would barge through the bathroom door asking if I was ok because he heard me weeping. I was trying to hide my tears, but I was too loud. Crying made me feel guilty for being sad about my child and her problems; a mother shouldn't feel that way about her child. It just continued the cycle.

I evaded public interactions as much as I could. I still went to church, but invitations for happy occasions like weddings or showers or parties would be met with excuses from me on why I couldn't attend. Not only that, I became great at avoiding people. I went to the stores right at opening or closing time, and sometimes 5 am when I thought my chances of seeing someone I knew was slim. All the avoidance was planned so I wouldn't have to have people question me about Jaycee's health status. I used drive-through options at the bank or a restaurant to decrease my social interactions as well. I went to great lengths to avoid people to prevent myself from hearing things that would upset me.

I wondered if anything good was going to happen to my family as my negativity was the only thing increasing at the time. It seemed like that first year of Jaycee's life was met with problem after problem and things weren't getting easier. I didn't know how to handle it mentally. During that time, if someone would have told me my house burned down and nothing was left, I would not have been surprised at all.

Christianity and depression aren't known for going together, but a Christian can be depressed. I tried so hard to fight the depression. I went to the altar to pray countless times with other, non-judgmental people from my church. Those women shed tears with me and offered the support I needed. At the end of the day, there was only one problem—I was left alone with my thoughts. That was something I had to take control of myself.

As time went on, I made the absolute worst choice in the depression battle. I stopped going forward at church and asking people to pray for me. I was embarrassed for my sadness about my child's problems and how I couldn't just get over them. But mainly, I believed a lie that kept popping in my head—everyone is tired of praying for you again. So, I worked to hide the pessimism and sorrow as best I could by faking smiles and saying I was fine.

But, I wasn't fine. I was far from fine. My actions and emotions said otherwise. I just didn't know how to help myself. I waited for the time when I would somehow supernaturally just become happy and make it through a couple of days in a row without crying. I believed this day would come on its own without me doing anything special. I was wrong.

I wasn't sad every moment of every day. Jaycee's soft skin, adorable face, and sweet noises were just heartwarming. She made me happy. I loved being her mom. It's very hard to explain how on the one hand I felt very lost and depressed and on the other hand I was happy being Jaycee's mom. I suppose all the stress of the unplanned problems and the fear of the unknown was just too much.

Through this depression, I became more and more lost in my faith. After I had Jaycee, so much changed in my professional and personal life. My faith had changed, too. I always believed God was a just God. He was a healer who loved and cared for us. God heard the prayers of believers and gave answers in one way or another.

Suddenly, I found myself being challenged in these ideas for the first time in my life. With my innocent daughter's health in jeopardy, it didn't seem like God was just at all. It really seemed unfair that I had faithfully served God and was now watching my child suffer. Instead of Jaycee being healed, she had to undergo a heart surgery and all the pain that goes with it. It didn't feel like God loved us at all. *Did He forget about us?* Every time a diagnosis was handed to Jaycee, it was just more proof that God wasn't around. He seemed so distant and I questioned if my prayers did anything.

While I didn't understand everything about God, I didn't give up completely. I knew I wouldn't always feel that way, that I needed time to develop a different perspective. I still went to church weekly and listened to Christian music. I still read my Bible and hung up scriptures around the house. I looked at my relationship with God as a marriage. I was committed to the end... in sickness or health, good times or bad. This was a bad time, but I wouldn't give up.

Though I didn't give up on God, I did give up my positions in the church. I didn't feel like I could minister to the youth when I felt so empty. I really should have given up the positions before I had Jaycee due to an unexplained feeling I had, but I didn't. When Jaycee was around 6 months old, I withdrew from all my positions. I felt bad about not being there for some of the youth that I had developed relationships with, but I had to focus on my family and my own mental health.

When Jaycee was around 10 months old, something started to change. I realized Jaycee would be a year old soon, which meant I was approaching nearly a year in an uncontrollable depression. Enough was enough. Though I know it is different for everyone suffering from depression, I knew I had to take my life back. I pushed myself and worked to get back to a better place.

I'm not sure what helped me get out of the deep pit of depression. For me, the biggest help was realizing that happiness wasn't going to just come to me; I had to decide to end the sadness

By: Evana Sandusky

and negative thoughts. If a song made me sad, I didn't listen to it. If a person tended to upset me, I guarded myself against that person instead of society as a whole. If I found something upsetting, I gave myself a day or two to react to it, and then moved on. I never sought medical intervention. One doctor recognized my struggles early on and offered medication as a treatment. I declined it thinking I was not that bad. I realize now that was a mistake, and I wish I would have listened to that doctor. I struggled for months and perhaps I would have gotten better faster had I gotten proper treatment.

By the time Jaycee's first birthday came, I had a genuine smile on my face. The depression was no longer controlling my days. I was learning to be in charge of it and was gaining ground. Was the depression completely gone forever? No. But I have never felt as sad and desperate as I did those first few months after Jaycee's birth and diagnoses. I have learned to recognize when I am going down the wrong emotional path, so I am able to make changes and seek support.

I had survived much in the first year of being Jaycee's mother. I was happy to be in a better place with my attitude and emotions, but my faith was still struggling. As I continued to serve God, there just didn't seem to be much of anything that made sense. I prayed for Jaycee to make progress and to stay healthy. But she didn't and wasn't going to.

It's hard to pray for someone with chronic medical conditions and maintain your faith. At some point in my walk with God, I went from praying hours a day to next to nothing. It wasn't a conscious decision; I just prayed less and less until there was nothing left of my prayer life.

There were many reasons why I didn't pray but none of them were good. The biggest thing that stopped me was my absolute confusion! People offered me their "biblical" perspective on my situation, frequently commenting: God gives special children to special parents because He knows they will raise them well; God makes people with Down syndrome and He chose you to care for her; or God never gives you more than you can handle. Those comments didn't help my Christianity at all. In fact, they ruined my relationship with God. I heard so many little comments about Jaycee, God, her life, and her future from people who meant well but didn't understand. They didn't know I was teetering on the edge of my faith wondering which way I would fall. These comments made me feel helpless about everything happening with Jaycee. They did not bring comfort in any way.

It's challenging to care for a child with medical issues and understand the bigger plan. Thus, I searched for the deeper spiritual meaning to it all. Where was God anyway? Why should I pray for Jaycee to get better if this is how God made her? Is it selfish of me to pray for Jaycee to thrive and not be delayed? Is that prayer for me or her? Where does disability fit in the Christian world?

I had so many questions and so many thoughts. I had given up trying to spiritually understand my situation with my beautiful daughter. I unconsciously decided it was easier to withdraw myself than fight through all the perplexities about which prayer was the "correct" one. I spent the first few years of her life being confused spiritually and not understanding God's perspective on my daughter.

Faith in God is the source of hope and peace; when I stopped praying, I had neither. I considered myself a Christian, as I continued going to church and believing in God, but I was not praying. I was lost and desperately needed spiritual help to make sense of my life and my faith.

The Faith Badge I earned by praying, fasting, and believing God was just after Jaycee's birth was in real disarray. In just a few years, my badge was ripped, tattered, and barely hanging on. I struggled to make sense of her health problems, surgeries, and health scares. I didn't know how to react to each event and how to be a person of faith in the situations I was finding myself in as Jaycee's mom. My Faith Badge needed mending!

A change had to be made. My husband and I felt the biggest thing to help us both would be to make a fresh start by attending a new church. If you have ever had to leave a church full of people you like, then you'd understand how hard it was to leave. Our church had always supported us with Jaycee. We knew switching churches would, in a way, isolate us even further. There would be no prayer chains started when Jaycee was sick, no more hospital visits from clergy, and no one generously preparing meals for us when we came home from a hospital admission. It was not an easy decision, but we felt it was what we needed to do.

When we decided to make this change, Jaycee was 4-years old and Elijah was just a year old. In my four years of being a parent, I had experienced my child needing the NICU, having two open heart surgeries and a couple of minor surgeries, getting several diagnoses, having a few hospital admissions, using home oxygen and a CPAP, and I had a miscarriage. In four years, my faith had been challenged, as well as my own emotional and mental well-being. Looking back, it was no wonder that I was struggling so much. Most parents don't experience what I had in a lifetime, let alone four years. Of course, my emotions were all over the place and I wasn't always able to see things with a healthy perspective. So, we left our comfort zone in a familiar church and looked for a place that would help me repair my Faith Badge.

We started attending a new church that was larger than we were accustomed to attending. We were a face in the crowd for quite a long time. It was hard to be "on our own," but I felt it was a good time of stretching for me. I needed to take back ownership of my faith. The sermons and the underlying messages at the church were just what we were looking for to get through the week.

I needed to hear that God was good even when things were bad. The reminder that just because you have faith doesn't mean all your fears disappear was imperative. Faith and staying positive required me to resist those adverse thoughts. I was reminded that God loves us, all of us. Jaycee's medical problems were not from God, though her spirit was God-created and she was important to Him. I needed to hear that life in general was a blessing, not that good health was a blessing. In short, I was reminded of things I had known all my life. I did, in fact, serve a just and loving God. This truth had been hidden by the pain caused by unexpected experiences over a few years.

The first time I walked into our new church I felt God strongly. I wanted to cry being in His presence again. The God I was seeking was there calling me to intensify my relationship with Him. I slowly began to trust God again. I had to confront my pains, my fears, my disappointments, and my distrust that had stemmed from seeing my daughter's life in jeopardy.

It turns out that our decision to change churches came at a critical time. A few months after starting the new church and understanding my faith again, Jaycee's battle with Wolff-Parkinson White syndrome started. I never would have survived those months when Jaycee's life was in peril without having the renewed spiritual life from our new church.

As the months and years passed, my Faith Badge became more securely attached. I came to an understanding that I didn't comprehend everything about God and my situation, but I loved Him anyway. I realized that when I stopped praying and talking to God, I did not allow a pathway of encouragement from Him. Adversity became under more control when I started to pray again.

I concluded being a Christian does not prevent trying events from occurring in our lives. I was spiritually immature in my faith when I believed God would spare me from any trials and sorrow in life. God is the person to run to when things on Earth aren't perfect; He is not the person to take your frustrations out on. I don't believe God's sole purpose is to protect Christians from vexing times; someone rooted in faith should not be swayed by any event, good or bad. After all, Heaven is the only perfect place where we will only experience good.

Once I discovered that truth, maintaining my Faith Badge was easier. I no longer viewed one of Jaycee's health crises as a sign God was not in our lives or that God didn't care. Now I saw it as an isolated event for God to give me the strength to pull through it. That perspective changed my life and helped me find real joy in less than ideal circumstances.

Over time, my Faith Badge was completely restored. I could pray for people again and more importantly I could pray for myself and Jaycee again. If someone was going through a difficult ordeal, I could find words of encouragement. It took work and effort over time, but things got back to normal. I understood why some parents, when faced with a tragedy with their child, lost all hope and gave up on God. When your child hurts, you hurt. I think it's hard to understand how God fits into all that hurt. Luckily, I did make sense of it all.

I am grateful my Faith Badge was restored. I have made a conscious decision to monitor its condition and never want it to get back to that battered state again.

By: Evana Sandusky

CHAPTER 12:

THE STRESS BADGE

Stress Badge: This badge is given to a mother who feels a complete and utter amount of pressure while caring for her child or dealing with issues related to her child. This badge is not necessarily one a mother tries to earn; instead, the mother finds this badge is automatically given when the effects of stress become evident in the mother's body or mental status. This badge can be earned or lost several times throughout motherhood.

Stress Badge Earned: 2006

Stress before getting pregnant was somewhat unknown to me. I managed my responsibilities in work, church ministry, and marriage well. I could relax easily and brush things off and let problems go. If someone asked me if I had ever felt stress, I could honestly answer no. That was all about to change in 2006.

Prior to having my difficult pregnancy with Jaycee, I had not experienced much in the way of tragedy or misfortune. I had caring, Christian parents and an older brother that I admired. I had a happy life. Of course, there were a few bumps in the road, but nothing had a major, long-term impact on me.

After becoming pregnant, I knew what stress was and I had more compassion for people dealing with it. I understood what it was like to have your thoughts consumed by your present situation. I knew thinking positive was not enough, nor was it easy, as stress manifests in a person's body if it occurs long enough.

Being pregnant with Jaycee was mentally tiring. When the spotting was heavy, I was consumed with worry, doubt, and stress. The sickness and nausea of the pregnancy wore me down over the months and added to my anxiety. But I was optimistic because once I was holding my newborn baby, I knew the Stress Badge would be gone forever.

Forever was a really long time. The reality was my Stress Badge became more affixed to my sash after Jaycee's birth. Caring for her, as I have already described in detail, was many things but stressful was the most accurate. *Was she eating enough? Was her congestive heart failure getting worse? Was I doing everything right?* I had many responsibilities with Jaycee's care and it made me feel overwhelmed. I found it was hard to just sit, relax, and be in the moment. I also had so many doubts; though some were valid, some were completely based off fear. For instance, I was always worried she would stop breathing in her sleep. I was plagued with the notion to check on Jaycee and recheck her when she was an infant sleeping in the bassinet.

After Jaycee's first open heart surgery and the end of her home oxygen use, the Stress Badge loosened up from my sash. Jaycee was around 8 months old at that time. Some of my fears and concerns were lessened thanks to her improvement in health. There was, for a time, fewer medications which was one less thing for me to keep track of each day. The threat of worsening congestive heart failure was nonexistent after surgery, which took quite a tremendous load off my mind. Jaycee was getting older and bigger, though she was still small for her age, but, she didn't look so fragile. She was more active, her personality was showing, and we had some fun and sweet times with her improved health.

The Stress Badge never left, but it did lose some threading over the next few months. It was still hard juggling Jaycee's frequent doctor appointments, my return to work after six months, and fitting in all of Jaycee's early intervention therapies and home activities. My stress was getting more manageable, which made me confident it would leave soon, as we weren't expecting any more hiccups with Jaycee's health.

Then the need came for Jaycee to have more medical tests, the second heart surgery, and additional medications with the diagnosis of asthma. A miscarriage further added to my life story as a mom and so my Stress Badge was tightly stitched back up.

"You are ok. You're handling all this well," I would tell myself. *Lies!* I wanted to believe, and I wanted to be fine.

I suppose I learned in time how to hide my stress well from others. By the time Jaycee was three, I was good at smiling through my busy stressful mind. I didn't want people to think Jaycee was a burden to me, as she wasn't. I was happy to do things for Jaycee as her mother, but it was tough at times. I was afraid if I was open about my concerns people would perceive me as a miserable person who hated her life. That wasn't the case, but I was stressed from the demands of life and afraid to show it. I didn't ask anyone for extra help, so I could have a day off from her care. I didn't ask therapists or doctors to decrease appointments because it was too much for me. I never shared with any of Jaycee's doctors that her care was becoming quite intense and ask for adjustments. I kept going along, adding more responsibilities to my parenting. I needed a break in some way and didn't or couldn't ask for one.

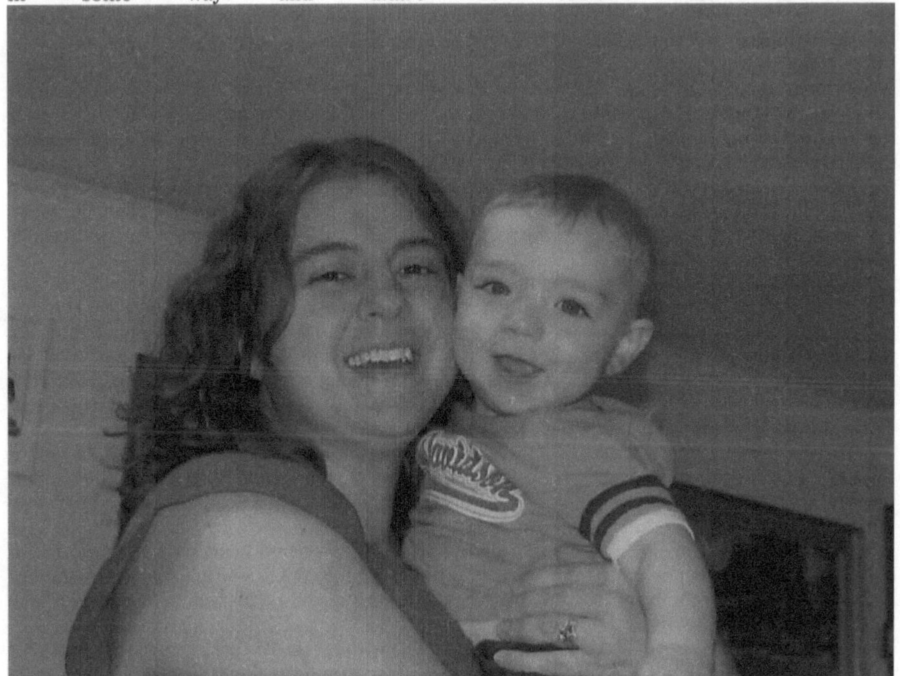

Elijah and Mommy in 2010

After Elijah was born, another layer of stress was added. I loved having a newborn son. He was an answered prayer. Jaycee loved her brother, too, (She still loves her brother) which wasn't always good. At three-and-a-half- years old, she wanted to pick him up but couldn't put him down gently. When Jaycee came home from school, I really had to watch Elijah like a hawk. Fixing supper became the time when Elijah was most vulnerable to an attack of love from Jaycee. I learned to keep him in a vibrating seat, a swing or some other infant contraption to prevent Jaycee

By: Evana Sandusky

from trying to move him, pick him up, or inadvertently hurt him. She didn't understand how fragile he was and it was stressful until he got bigger and learned how to walk—sometimes right away from her!

To my credit, there were moments when the Stress Badge was off or just barely hanging on. There were great days and weeks when the stress wasn't there. I don't know how it happened though I found myself enjoying my family and completing my work without thinking too much about Jaycee's health issues or her at-home treatments. There were times the routine and schedule seemed easier and I had free time to relax and let life flow. I didn't think about what task I had to do next or how I would get it all done or even dread an upcoming appointment on the calendar. I was doing well. I couldn't predict how long the Stress Badge would be gone, but I enjoyed the times when it was absent.

My life as a mother eventually fell into a routine. Our life was our version of normal and it was nice to have some peaceful moments. Then without warning, as quickly as the badge disappeared, it would return with a health event or diagnosis or problem. It seemed the stress was out of my control and it was impossible to keep away for long amounts of time. I didn't know how to manage the stress for years, and it got worse before it got better.

It was at its absolute highest during the months between Jaycee's diagnosis of Wolff-Parkinson White syndrome and her two heart ablations. That Stress Badge was super-glued to me at that time. I prayed and believed Jaycee would be fine, but I was constantly being challenged that something might cause her WPW to trigger. It's difficult to carry on with life with such information.

I slowly recognized some signs of my manifesting stress. Around each of Jaycee's heart surgeries, my stress was expressed by snapping at my poor husband or getting way too upset over the slightest thing. I had trouble sleeping and never felt relaxed, but the stress was more internalized during Jaycee's scare with WPW.

I went through the motions of my everyday life but in the back of my mind, I was *constantly* thinking about Jaycee. If she was at school, I wondered if her heart was ok at that moment. Jason and I did not catch her tachycardia immediately the first time, so I could not be assured her teachers at school would either.

When Jaycee's first heart ablation for WPW was completed, the Stress Badge suddenly left my sash. I felt such relief! I knew I was carrying quite a mental load and stress while Jaycee was in the danger zone, but I wasn't fully aware of it until the relief set in. I had really been weighed down by the threat of Jaycee's life ending at any moment, which made it difficult to enjoy any part of life or make long-term plans. It had all changed when the doctor announced it was successful. I remember sitting in the hospital room thinking all our lives would return to normal. I reflexively smiled for the first time in a long time. Jaycee would be fine; my daughter would be okay.

The badge came immediately back on me a month later when the WPW showed back up on the EKG. I was stunned when we were told Jaycee would need a second heart ablation. I wanted to deny it. This time the chances of her WPW firing again and causing death was slim, but it was still there.

The stress was back as Jaycee would have to undergo a second heart catheterization with ablation, but it couldn't be done immediately. A few more months of waiting would provide her body time to recuperate from the first ablation and allow more time for that Stress Badge to be sewed on more firmly.

I didn't want it to be this way. I didn't want to live with stress. At that time, I was caring for Jaycee and her toddling brother. I wanted to enjoy this time in my children's lives. There were times of joy, but stress was *always* an ugly feeling trying to steal away the faith and happiness that should have been more present. Like a ringing in my ears, stress was something in my life that, try as I could, I just couldn't ignore. I loved Jaycee so much and couldn't handle these health conditions that threatened her life.

Fortunately, the second ablation ended in success. WPW is just a note on Jaycee's health history, and the stress that came from that diagnosis and possible threats were gone. The ablation took place about a week before Elijah's second birthday. I truly had something to celebrate that day!

The WPW diagnosis understandably brought stress into my life. But even with it gone, I found the Stress Badge was just not ever leaving anymore. I had been too traumatized as a mother and it was all catching up with me. Denying that stress wasn't there or that I was "handling" it well just made it stick stronger.

One day, the stress couldn't be ignored. In the winter of 2012, I noticed my arms had a pins and needles feeling much like what people describe as their limb falling asleep. My neck muscles were incredibly tight as well. Try as I might, I could not roll my head around in a complete circle. I didn't know what was going on with my body and downplayed my symptoms until I could no longer ignore how I was feeling. I could not sleep on my side because my arms would fall asleep and wake me up. I couldn't hold an object like a telephone up to my ear for very long without my hand going numb briefly. Then my left hand became constantly numb. I couldn't type or use my left hand for much of anything without extreme pain. Once, I went through a fast food drive-thru grabbing the Styrofoam cup with my left hand. Unable to judge my grip, I squeezed the cup too hard, popped off the lid, and spilled some of the liquid sweetness all over me. Spilling soda on myself was the breaking point. I had to see what was wrong with me.

I eventually had to make a doctor's appointment for myself, which was something I was not accustomed to doing. I sat in the doctor's office wondering what could be wrong with me. Even though it seems clear to me now, at the time I had truly no idea that stress was finally having an impact on my body. I blamed my symptoms on my continued need to lift Jaycee at times, who was now getting older and heavier. I even blamed my career choice for which I carried totes of therapy supplies around and then sat on the floor for hours a week doing speech therapy. I couldn't imagine at the time that my problems were from stress.

Some medications and wrist guards were prescribed but gave no relief. A couple of months later, I found myself at a specialist who gave me a diagnosis explaining all my symptoms but not the cause. The management included a variety of shoulder, arm, and chest stretches to relax my muscles. To learn these, I was given one appointment with a physical therapist. She pointed out to me that I always had my shoulders slightly hunched up. I had no idea my body was doing this! I left the appointment with a booklet of exercises to continue at home and more awareness of my body.

At home, I researched my diagnosis looking for more answers and possible treatments. I started doing the stretches at home and found them difficult since my muscles were incredibly tight and tense. I had to make a conscious effort throughout the day to lower my shoulders; I charged Jason with the task of pointing out my raised shoulders when he saw me doing it at home, which ended up being quite often at first.

It was at that point when I decided to give massage therapy a try. I had never had a massage because the idea never appealed to me. I don't particularly like having people touch me, so I was afraid I would be too tense to reap any benefits. Bravely, I entered a massage room with probably as much anxiety as when I go to the dentist. The pain and the numbness in my arm and hands reminded me that I needed to give it a try. It turned out the hour on that massage table was not as bad as I had pictured. During the massage, I became aware of the knots and tightness in my muscles, which helped me so much. *I didn't realize my body was that tight!*

I became a massage therapy addict for a short time. It can be a very expensive addiction though as I went once a week for a few months. Lying on the table, I concentrated on my body, something I hadn't done in a long time. I was accustomed to being busy *every second*. I realized just how much I had been taxing my body and how difficult it was for me to just sit and relax. The massages forced me to stop and try to clear my head and see that I needed to try to carve out times of rest at home, too.

I started to get better, but I was still unclear as to why my muscles were tight. I blamed much of it on that-years of lifting my growing child. One of the massage therapists asked me a few standard small-talk questions at one of my sessions. For whatever reason, I mentioned Jaycee had special needs and required a lot of medical interventions.

She made just one comment, "That must be stressful."

I answered her with an honest, "Yes," which got me thinking.

By: Evana Sandusky

A lightbulb started to slowly grow brighter and brighter. *Could all my symptoms be from stress?* The doctor didn't think so, but I continued to read and look for answers. I had to take a good, hard look at myself—I was more stressed out than I was willing to admit.

As my symptoms eased up and the pins and needles in my hand went away, I was grateful the treatment was working. A few months into my regimen, Jaycee went into the ICU. It was during her hospital stay that I positively identified the link between my stress and the effect it was having on my muscles and body as the numbness returned to my hand. There was no denying my physical issues were a result of the stress I was under. I couldn't get a medical doctor to agree with me, but that is fine as I live in this body and know how it reacts in stressful moments.

As the stress to my body became clear, I knew I had to somehow reduce my stress level. Jaycee's care required certain things of me every day. When she was sick, the care rose to another intense level. As her situation was not going to change any time soon, I had to do something to try to stop stress from breaking my body even more.

I knew I needed to reduce my stress, but I didn't know how to do it in order to change or where to begin. I made some small changes that helped me little by little. I found when I made forward progress by starting an exercise or stretching routine, an illness would wreak havoc on my routine and send all my good habits away. Then I would have to start all over.

The Stress Badge was never something I intended to have on my sash, but it happened. I would like to deny the Stress Badge ever took up residence in my mothering journey, but it did. I just wish in retrospect that I would have caught it early on or not lied to myself by repeatedly convincing myself, "I'm fine. I'm handling this well." If only I would have viewed some of Jaycee's scary health issues as traumas for myself too, perhaps I could have accepted the fact that I needed help also. Plus, if only a doctor who knew Jaycee's or my story would have asked me how I really was—from the ICU to the doctor after my miscarriage—not one professional sat down and talked with me about my stress related to Jaycee's condition or my own. It doesn't seem to be an area that's addressed often for parents, but hopefully one day it will be.

I love my daughter and want nothing more than for her to live a full and long life. That desire feels threatened in a health crisis and my body's reaction is added stress. Jaycee isn't stressful—I want to make that clear. But it is stressful when I am responsible for keeping her healthy (i.e. making sure her medications are given properly or her breathing isn't labored) and when, despite my best efforts, she needs to go the hospital for care. Prior to 2006, I didn't comprehend a stressful life. Now, I know that life all too well.

Today, I am sorry to say the Stress Badge is probably on my sash more than it is off. Through all of Jaycee's emergency room runs, ICU scares, surgeries, and diagnoses, my body became conditioned to an uptight state. I'm still trying to loosen up the grip the stress had placed on me. My hand rarely gets numb anymore unless Jaycee's in the hospital or ill. I still get tight muscles in my neck, shoulders, and arms, which I feel is a pretty good indication that I am still in this battle. I do try to listen to my body and do things for myself to ease my tightness. I have not figured out how to conquer this badge and rip it off, but I hope and pray that one day I will have a solution.

CHAPTER 13:

THE SECURITY BADGE

> *Security Badge: This badge is given to a mother who learns how to keep her child safe and secure beyond the usual and typical need. Moms earn this badge when they typically find their child wandering off in public places or trying to leave the house without consent. Moms in these situations must take added precautions to keep their child safe. This badge can be earned only one time per child after a successful system is in place.*

Security Badge Earned: 2009

I was warned by other parents: "Once she starts walking, you won't be so happy."

Not me, I thought. I will be happy to finally see Jaycee walking. At 20 months, she had started toddling a few steps independently. I was looking forward to having her walk with me instead of carrying her everywhere.

It was true though. As she got better at walking, I had my regrets! Safety became priority number one. I had to intensify the lockdown procedures at home and in public.

At home, Jaycee was into everything!! Anything she could reach from her short two-year-old stature, she did, and it was pulled to the ground. While she thought exploring and throwing things around was fun, she had little understanding of what she was doing. Concepts like if something was hot or could hurt her were foreign to Jaycee. She didn't really understand the word "no" that well either, even though I said it often.

We started with the normal safety precautions—kitchen cabinet locks, a baby gate positioned on the upstairs steps, and a door knob cover on the door leading to the basement. But these typical baby-proofing actions weren't enough to keep Jaycee safe.

I had to come up with other measures to ensure protection when she was home. I put pony tail holders on furniture two knobs close together to kept her from opening them; a lock was placed up high on her closet door where I kept all her medical supplies; and doors to rooms Jaycee didn't need to be in were always kept shut—always! The bathroom door was always shut because if she got in, she would be in the trashcan or unrolling the toilet paper. The front door leading to outside was always closed and locked to prevent her from going outside on her own. She couldn't open the doors for quite a while, so this worked well for a few years.

When we moved Jaycee into a toddler bed, safety at night became an issue. We would wake up in the morning and find Jaycee asleep in the hallway or on the living room floor and found the refrigerator door slightly ajar more than once. Even though we used baby monitors, she quietly left her room undetected by us though we still woke up to find our nonverbal toddler asleep where she shouldn't be. We worried about her safety.

The solution became to put a baby gate in front of Jaycee's bedroom door at night before we went to bed. Jaycee's room was safe as there were no dangers within her reach, so we felt this was the best and safest option to try. We also felt in an emergency at night, we would know exactly where Jaycee was. There were times we woke to find Jaycee asleep next to her baby gate in her room, but this slowly stopped as she realized she had nowhere to go. Really, the gate seemed to help her understand to stay in her room, and eventually it was no longer needed.

During Jaycee's toddler and pre-school years, I felt my life at home revolved around locks and gates. Sometimes I second-guessed what I was doing, thinking perhaps I was restricting her too much in some ways. Now I realize it was all necessary. When she understood how to safely navigate the house, safety measures were slowly stripped away. The day we were able to finally rid ourselves of baby gates was an exciting day for us!

Around age 6, Jaycee's needs changed slightly. She was older and stronger, but she still didn't understand dangers outside the house. Jaycee couldn't ask me to go outside and I don't think she gave getting permission any thought. She didn't seem to connect behavior with consequences either, making it hard for her to understand why she was in trouble. Jaycee's favorite activity was swinging on our playground, but it sometimes made her try to escape the house. Fortunately, we don't live on a busy street, but we do have a pool in the backyard. I was very paranoid about Jaycee doing something that would put herself in danger.

Extra measures were put in place on two of the doors leading outside—a dead bolt and a pool lock. Jason made sure to put a lock high up on the door that led to the pool, so Jaycee couldn't reach it. I also made stop signs with the words, "Ask Mom" that were placed on two of the doors. I had my doubts about the signs, but the visual cue seemed to help her remember to wait on me before going outside. At first, I was reluctant to place the stop signs in the house; my house isn't fancy, but the signs seemed tacky. Still, I had to look beyond some of my preferences and do what might possibly help Jaycee.

Besides finding ways to keep Jaycee safe at home, I earned my Security Badge while keeping Jaycee safe in public. My husband and I tried to give Jaycee some freedom as a toddler and allow her to walk with us in public; however, she would always let go of our hands and run off, laughing and giggling loudly as she ran away. She thought it was the best time ever! But we did not!

From the moment we took her out in public, she never wanted to stay with us. I recall reading about this problem in the Down syndrome population in an article around that time. One article stated children usually outgrew this behavior at age nine. My first thought was, *how many years did I have left of this?* I felt hopeless in being able to change this behavior quickly. It was challenging helping a toddler with an intellectual disability who only said a couple of words understand the importance of staying with us in public.

Then the day came when I purchased one of those dreaded child leashes. Gasp! I always thought parents who used those looked foolish yet there I was joining them. Sometimes the very thing you say you will never do as a parent comes back to haunt you. I felt so self-conscious using the toddler leash in public, but it was necessary because Jaycee wandered off so much. So, I became a leash parent. I could grab hold of Jaycee's leash when she let go of my hand. The leash was a good back up measure to keep her with me. It helped at certain events like parades when she needed to stay in one spot but have a little freedom. We used them in stores or other outings where we knew she would have a desire to explore but possibly run off, which was almost everywhere we went.

There was one big problem with the leash. It really frustrated Jaycee. It gave us peace of mind, but it made her mad. She would plop down and scream and cry because she wanted to go somewhere and couldn't. I was spared the fun of chasing after a child in a store with the leash, but I encountered the new experience of dealing with a complete meltdown. She just did not understand what was going on.

Jaycee's behaviors out in public became a gamble. Will she run off? Should I use the leash? Will this cause a complete meltdown? I didn't really know what to do though I knew her running off was a problem. Early on I could catch her easily, pick her up, and place her in a stroller or shopping cart. The leash was a quick solution and one that minimized the stress while in public.

Eventually, Jaycee outgrew the leashes and I focused on containment in public. This meant using strollers or shopping carts. The day Jaycee got too big for the child's seat in a shopping cart was disappointing. I had a new problem. If I put her down, she would run off. If I placed her "illegally" in the shopping cart with my groceries, she would throw them out of the cart. Jaycee got a thrill of watching things go out of the cart and onto the floor. After a few messes in the store, I deemed the regular shopping cart was no longer an option for her.

Next solution? I was fortunate to find a few stores near me that had child seated shopping carts or shopping carts with a car attached to the front. There were only a couple of stores with these special carts that I could shop at with her though. Plus, I had to pray the carts were available when I got to the store! These carts were my next best options when I had to shop with Jaycee. By that time, I was trying to go shopping while she was in pre-school, so I could reduce the stress of an outing. Sometimes, it was unavoidable though. For the most part, these were good options, however, Jaycee could get out of the toy car part of the shopping cart and a chase would soon start.

Shopping with her in those car carts required me to be very observant and on guard. I couldn't causally stroll through the store. I was a focused and alert woman on a mission. God help me if someone I knew in the store saw me and wanted to chat. I was on the clock with Jaycee. Five minutes chit-chatting with a friend was five more minutes added to our time in the store and increasing the likelihood of a running issue.

Eventually, there came a sad day when Jaycee was still running off in public but outgrew all our options. When I took Jaycee and Elijah out in public alone, I had to think about every move I made, especially keys in hand before walking to my vehicle. One second of letting go of her hand to retrieve my keys from my purse was enough time for Jaycee to dart away. If we were walking towards my vehicle, she would typically run to it, but she was unaware of other vehicles in a parking lot that may be moving about. No matter how many times I said no, it didn't click with her. She just could not comprehend the concept, which put me on guard more knowing she could get hurt or I'd lose her. I was like her Secret Service detail always trying to be a step ahead to protect my asset.

When Jason or my mother accompanied me on trips, one person would be designated the keeper, so to speak. Jaycee's keeper engaged her in public and kept a hand (and eye) on her always. Going out with another adult allowed me to relax a bit. I could even pay at the store without trying to keep tabs on Jaycee. Yes, every second mattered.

By chance, I encountered a man at a speech therapy conference whose profession was durable medical equipment. I questioned him about getting Jaycee a stroller. I wasn't even sure they made strollers for older children since I knew they weren't in stores, but did they exist anywhere? He informed me these strollers did exist and with Jaycee's medical diagnoses, she would most likely get one from our insurance.

After that, I decided Jaycee needed to get a medical stroller. It took a few months from start to finish, but soon Jaycee was sitting in her new green stroller. It was a blessing to have something for Jaycee! We could take her places that required walking long distances, like malls or zoos, without the fear of what we would do if she decided to meltdown or run off. I now had a way to contain her again, and I was so grateful.

One day, I made the very brave decision to try to go grocery shopping with Jaycee in her stroller by myself. I felt nervous and scared as I unloaded her stroller in the Wal-Mart parking lot. Inside the store, I grabbed a shopping cart; pushing Jaycee's stroller in front of me and pulling the shopping cart behind me, I felt awkward maneuvering both around the store. More than once, I rammed Jaycee's stroller or the cart into shelving. I felt very self-conscious and believed everyone I passed by was looking at this very long train of stroller-cart combination. I made it through the shopping experience tired but satisfied this was a good option for us. Jaycee was content to sit in her stroller and I was happy to be able to get groceries with my children with little stress, as Elijah could sit in the cart or be trusted to walk beside me.

Over time, I became a pro at shopping in this manner. I'm no longer self-conscious; if people stare, it doesn't bother me. Elijah eventually got big enough to push his sister, making the shopping experience a little easier, too. Years later when Jaycee outgrew her stroller we got a wheelchair for her, which was needed more for health and stamina reasons rather than security ones.

As Jaycee has gotten older, the need to keep her safe is still there, but it is not nearly as intense. Her limited verbal speech and difficulty comprehending dangers continue to keep me refining my skills for the Security Badge. It was around age 9 or 10 that she stopped running off in public just like that article predicted all those years ago. Thank God that stage is over! Still, I do have to pay attention in crowds or public places because I don't want to get separated from my daughter who cannot say her own name clearly or give out basic information.

Looking back, I can see I made many errors while trying to keep my Security Badge when Jaycee was between 2-5 years old. She did not understand much about her safety, but I didn't do enough to help her understand. I wish I would have used more visuals and not just picked her up and moved her when she melted down on the floor refusing to move. Picking her up and moving

By: Evana Sandusky

her where I wanted only hurt me in the long run. When all eyes seem to be on you and your child in public, it's hard to know how to respond and think of long term consequences.

Despite the mistakes I have made, I do feel I did many things well for Jaycee. Earning a Security Badge has taken patience, thinking, reasoning, creativeness, and trial-and-error. Helping a child understand safety is a very difficult task. We have escaped any major disasters, so in that respect we have been successful.

CHAPTER 14:

THE HANDICAP PLACARD BADGE

> *Handicap Placard Badge: This badge is awarded to the mother who must obtain and use a handicap placard for their vehicle while transporting her child with medical needs or developmental needs. This badge can only be earned once for each child.*

Handicap Placard Badge Earned: 2013

From the moment Jaycee was a day old, she was labeled. The only time I didn't associate a diagnosis with her was while I was pregnant. Over the years, I have seen Jaycee's name attached to many reports, medical documents, and special education forms. Still, the day I asked her doctor if she qualified for a handicap placard, I felt odd. This was going to be a new situation for us. If she qualified, I was literally going to hang a sign that announced someone exiting my van had a disability. I wasn't entirely sure how I felt about that.

Even though nothing had changed with Jaycee, applying for this permit was a little emotional for me; I never expected this for my child. I felt like I was achieving a new level of acceptance by admitting the fact that Jaycee's medical and developmental issues were impacting us more than most people realized.

Based upon her lung and heart issues, Jaycee was eligible for the handicap placard. I was grateful for this for so many reasons. If I was taking her to the store in one of my push-the-stroller-pull-the-cart trips, I could park a little closer. When the weather was extremely hot and humid or icy cold, I could park her closer to buildings to lessen her time outside.

The biggest reason for trying to obtain the handicap placard at that time in Jaycee's life was we were planning a family vacation to Walt Disney World the following year. We felt in the place that required so much walking, this would be a real benefit to us.

The doctor and I filled out the required documents to send in to the state for approval. The placard came in the mail several weeks later while Jaycee was in the hospital on the ventilator during her bad illness in 2013. Talk about good timing! When Jaycee left the hospital, she was not walking on her own due to muscle loss, so it was a blessing to have the placard during all the trips to her rehabilitation therapy and when going out until her stamina improved.

Having the placard was such a benefit for Jaycee. At the time, she had already had two heart surgeries, two heart ablations, battled asthma frequently, completed twice daily vest airway clearance treatments, used a BiPAP at night for four years, and been diagnosed with a lung cyst. Her heart and lung problems impacted her daily life; however, those issues were unseen by people who observed a child exiting a vehicle parked in a handicap spot. There were times when I felt the stares of people as we walked away from or towards our legally parked vehicle. People were focused on me and never gave a thought to the fact a child in the vehicle owned the placard. Whenever I used Jaycee's stroller, I rarely get a strange look in the parking space as it is the type of visual people are searching for when making those mental judgements on who or who does not deserve to use such a space.

I admit I have had those moments of judgment, too. I see someone who looks completely able-bodied using a placard that may belong to someone else. Even though I have questioned some people in my mind, I have never approached anyone, as I never felt it was my place to call someone out publicly. That was between the person and his or her conscience; unfortunately, other people are not like me.

For example, one Saturday afternoon I decided to take the kids grocery shopping. I try to avoid Saturdays because they tend to be busy and crowded. On that day, I would be doing my stroller and cart method of shopping in a very popular store. When we pulled into the parking lot I was glad there was a handicap parking spot available for us. Before we exited the vehicle, I hung the placard and said a silent prayer that this trip in the store would be a peaceful one.

Jaycee did great in the store. She didn't get out of her stroller and run away nor swipe things off the shelf or throw things on the floor. Elijah, a first grader at the time, was helping me load things into the cart. As I placed the groceries and Jaycee's stroller in the back of my van, I thought about how wonderful this shopping trip went. Sometimes, they were stressful, but that day was not until...

Jaycee and I climbed into the vehicle at the same time. As I buckled up, a man tapped on my window. I partially rolled it down to see if he needed help—he didn't.

"I don't know how you got that handicap placard, but obviously, you don't need it," said the elderly man wearing a large cowboy hat.

"It's not mine. It's my daughter's. She has Down syndrome and lots of health problems," I replied in a shaky voice. Subsequently, I rolled my daughter's window down for him to view the person in question as if I needed his approval.

"Well, you can park here then. But I saw you get in your van so nimbly that I knew you couldn't be disabled. My wife is disabled. She needs these spaces. You would not believe how many people use these illegally, so I watch for people who shouldn't be using them," said the self-proclaimed sheriff of the grocery store parking lot.

He then questioned if Jaycee had ever exited the vehicle, since he didn't see her get inside the van. That was laughable. Like I could really go shopping for 45 minutes in a store and leave her to sit in a vehicle alone. Never! Hence, the previous chapter on the Security Badge.

At that point, I reminded him I had legally been issued the placard and reiterated that my daughter has been in the hospital multiple times for heart and lung issues. I found myself playing with the power windows out of nervousness, not quite knowing if I should roll my window up and cut him off or roll it down farther. The man continued his speech that he has probably given to other people about how wrong it is to park illegally. He tried to get me to agree with him, that abuse of these parking spots is common, but I didn't know how to respond. Frankly, I was ready to take my children home and forget I had this conversation with this guy who ruined what was a nice outing for us.

When I could tell he was not going to make a heartfelt apology for his mistake and was going to continue his discourse on parking misuse, I decided it was time for me to leave. I stated again, "But I'm legal," rolled up my window, and drove off.

It was an odd feeling being wrongly accused of something. I don't respond well in heated situations, and it is only after the fact that I think of a thousand things to say, but during the situation I am rendered speechless. I wish I could have told that man more of Jaycee's story to help him understand that children go through unimaginable health issues making them eligible for this placard. Of course, my husband came up with the best question later—why wasn't the man inside the store helping his wife with a disability instead of in the parking lot confronting innocent people?

I drove off from the store having to regain my composure. *What just happened?* That is exactly what I asked myself when Elijah asked it out loud. My son, who was 6-years old at the time, had been listening to our conversation. I had to explain to him how the man thought I was doing something wrong. We have always openly talked about disabilities and illnesses. He could understand my explanation of the situation.

I drove a few miles down the road to pick up pizzas for supper but did not park in a handicap spot, opting a regular spot next to the handicap one. I sat in the van for a second while my hands finished shaking and took some deep breaths before taking the children in to order pizza. I could not believe what had just happened to me. A stranger tapping on my window and questioning my character had left me upset.

I had read stories of people finding nasty notes left on their car windshields making accusations of misuse of handicapped parking spots. Honestly, I was waiting for that to happen to me at some point, but I never imagined a face-to-face confrontation. On a positive note, I could defend myself and help the man understand nothing was improper about my actions. I hope my encounter taught him something about his approach and he makes a kinder, more inquisitive style the next time he decides to confront someone since **he** may be the one in the wrong. To date, I am thankful that was our one and only confrontation over my use of the handicap placard.

This badge brought mixed emotions for me. I was sorry my child needed it in the first place but happy it made some of our outings easier. I was apprehensive people would think Jaycee didn't deserve the placard and upset and angry when a man accused me of misuse. However, this badge, with all its unexpected emotions and situations, has brought a new perspective to this mothering experience for me.

By: Evana Sandusky

CHAPTER 15:
THE I.E.P. BADGE

I.E.P. Badge: This badge is awarded to a mother whose child has an Individualized Education Program (I.E.P.) to receive any special education service. This badge represents the hours spent attending meetings, reading paperwork, hearing diagnostic information, and making adjustments at home to help her child succeed in school. This badge can be awarded once for each mother's child.

I.E.P. Badge Earned: 2009

My child is going to need special education.

This thought ran around in my head more often than you would think soon after Jaycee was born. While I was adjusting to her diagnosis and worrying about her congestive heart failure when we brought her home from the hospital, I also grieved for the life that seemed to be set before her.

When you are told your child has Down syndrome, you are also told almost everything that goes along with it—developmental delays, difficulty speaking, and an intellectual disability. It would take a miracle for Jaycee to develop appropriately and achieve the things most parents assumed their child would automatically do. The future that everyone pictures their child having was taken away and ripped up for me the day the NICU doctor described my daughter's problems.

As soon as she was diagnosed, I had a picture of what Jaycee's life would be like down the road. In my profession, I had worked with children with special needs; many of their faces and struggles came to mind when I thought about Jaycee's educational future.

When your child is born with a diagnosis, things are different. You instantly question some of those big dreams and goals you instinctively have for your child. I wasn't sure if Jaycee would grow up to live independently, go to college, get married, or have a job. These events didn't seem like automatic possibilities anymore.

If your child is born healthy and typically developing, you have time to adjust to issues that come up. You develop a bond with your child, get to know his or her personality. As time goes on, it may be clear that your child may have weaknesses in an area, however, you can also see the strong points in his or her lives, too, and find a balance. It's harder when you are only told about your baby's problems and deficits because the balance gets thrown off.

For me, I have always known an I.E.P. would be in Jaycee's future since she was diagnosed. I suppose some people would say I was completely pessimistic from the start, but I prefer realistic. Before I had Jaycee, I worked in a school setting as a speech-language pathologist treating children and writing I.E.Ps. After working with so many children with diagnoses, my brain tied my past experiences to my daughter.

Prior to Jaycee being three years old and receiving an I.E.P., she had gone through our state's birth-3 program, which provides therapy services in the home for children with delays or developmental disabilities. By the time Jaycee ended the program, she was getting five hours weekly of speech, developmental, physical, and occupational therapy. These therapists and I met every six months to form an Individualized Family Service Plan (IFSP), or the equivalent of an I.E.P. up to age three, but it felt entirely different. Meetings were in my home and casual. As the parent, I was considered a vital part of the team determining Jaycee's top needs and had a major say in what services were provided to help Jaycee and our family. The goals were written in a family-friendly style with functional, routine-based skills at the core of what was addressed. Though I accepted these therapies and needs, I dreaded the day when Jaycee turned three and had to leave this program.

By the time Jaycee turned 3, I accepted the fact she would receive an I.E.P. and attend a special education classroom. Let's face it, no one wants his or her child to be in a special education classroom; it's not an easy thing to accept. You don't want your child to struggle or to be separated from typical peers. You don't want to walk your child into the room that everyone knows is for the "special kids," again labeling the child even more. You don't want your child's school life to start off in special education but sometimes, you must do the very thing you don't want to because it's what is best. It was necessary for Jaycee.

Just before Jaycee's 3rd birthday, I walked into the pre-school she would soon be attending for our first school meeting. The last time I had left this building I was carrying out my personal objects from the job I quit to care for Jaycee. Now, I was returning to find out how they would care for Jaycee. Even though I knew what was going to happen at the meeting, I had a sick feeling and wanted to throw up. I nervously wished none of this was happening. But, I put on a brave face and tried to act like I was fine, even though inside I was a mess.

This was going to be a big change for us. I knew what an I.E.P. and school would mean—Jaycee would no longer spend her days at home with me. I would no longer be watching and participating in therapy sessions or have the same opportunities to talk with Jaycee's therapists to brainstorm about problems that came up at home. I would not see first-hand what she was doing and have a chance to celebrate achievements with these people. Educational goals would be the priority and I would no longer be the *most* important member of Jaycee's team. It wasn't because Jaycee's school was "bad," it was just the way the education system operated.

As I approached the school, I inhaled deeply and soon took my place at the large conference table. Jaycee was with me, which helped me feel more at ease. The team discussed Jaycee's current levels of abilities in different areas and considered some of her challenges and things that needed addressing. Everyone was kind and respectful at the first I.E.P. meeting. Therapy services would be continued at the school. She would enter an early childhood classroom, which is a special classroom for children with delays or diagnoses. Some parents don't like these programs, but I had no problem with it. The teacher was trained to educate a child like mine, the class size was smaller, the instruction was more individualized, and the class utilized materials that would benefit Jaycee. At my suggestion, she would start off a few days a week for the remainder of the school year (three months) and then start full-time in the fall. I was happy the school agreed to this plan since it allowed her to slowly integrate into the school system while giving me a few more months with her at home.

Even though the meeting went well, the birth-3 documentation, meetings, and plan felt very different from the school's I.E.P. process. It is, for the most part, official and not family-friendly thanks to all of the mandates involved. It was page after page of information about the child and, in some ways, I felt glad my previous job had prepared me for that moment.

Besides the documentation, the school meeting was more structured and formal. There were a couple of people typing away intently on computers recording information. There was no discussion of "What's a concern of yours at home?" It didn't matter what was happening at home, as Jaycee's needs were now educationally focused. The questions centered on what she needed to do to function at school. There was a spot on the I.E.P. for parental input where some of the things and concerns I said in the meeting were recorded. I was most worried about Jaycee's safety, as at that time she was still prone to running off. She was also not feeding herself or talking, so those were concerns too. They were pleased to know she could identify several shapes and could label in sign language many animals, foods, and colors.

During the meeting, Jaycee was taken to the classroom to play while we spoke until she was brought back when the meeting was over. Jaycee, being social, interacted with the staff around the room. For some reason, she took part of her shirt and pulled it over her head exposing her belly. We all chuckled at Jaycee while she showed off her ability to partially undress herself.

With Jaycee's I.E.P. in my hand, I left the school with mixed emotions. The school and her placement would be good for her, still, it was a reality check to see MY child's name on an I.E.P.

By: Evana Sandusky

Before long, the details of the paperwork were put into motion, and the I.E.P. Badge was on me. My nonverbal, developmentally delayed, diaper-wearing, little girl would be starting pre-school on her third birthday. For the first time, she would be surrounded by people she didn't know. Jaycee had never been watched by anyone besides her grandparents and aunt. Even though I personally knew the people who would be working with Jaycee at the school, I was still leery. Letting go of your child, even if you know he or she will be in good hands, is very difficult when they have always been with you.

Most parents get upset when they walk their child to school for the first time—I was no different. In fact, all of Jaycee's special needs made it even harder for me. Jaycee knew hundreds of signs, far more than anyone that worked there, and some of her signs and gestures were only known by me. I was worried about her ability to communicate to other people and how she was unable to communicate most of her day to me when school was over. I learned how letting your child with large delays attend a new school takes a new kind of courage as a mother.

I bravely walked Jaycee into school, kissed her goodbye, and watched her take her first steps inside her new classroom. She was happy—too happy actually! There was no tearful goodbye that I was expecting (That happened on the second and third days instead!). So, I took myself to McDonald's for breakfast before setting off to work. I do recall watching the clock more than usual that day as I couldn't wait to pick Jaycee up and hear what she did at school.

Things have changed for me since the first I.E.P. meeting. I rarely get a stomachache before the meetings now. I know those in attendance well and I am not afraid to ask questions or give my input. The older Jaycee gets, the more aware I am of her abilities and limitations; therefore, the professionals weren't really telling me too many things to surprise me. For the most part, the school and I have agreed on what she needs for her education. I don't really have a horror story to tell like I have heard from so many other people and for that I'm thankful. The I.E.P. process is what is—not family-friendly—but I have gotten accustomed to the fact that Jaycee will need one while she is in school. I'm glad there's a system in place to help children like her because she has certainly benefited from these programs. I hope our experiences remain positive as she continues through school.

I.E.P. Badge Earned: 2013

Jaycee's I.E.P. was always anticipated and was no surprise to me. When my second child, Elijah, needed an I.E.P., it was completely unexpected.

Elijah was developing typically as a baby. When he was two, I became concerned his feet were turning in when he walked, and he often tripped when he tried to run. In fact, he really couldn't run because of it. Elijah had a tricycle but didn't seem to have the muscle strength to pedal it. He always sat with his legs making a "W" shape on the floor and often slept and sat on his knees, too. These problems were just minor issues compared to what I dealt with for Jaycee, which was why they were easy to dismiss at first.

I watched Elijah's progress for a while and discussed the physical and muscle concerns with my husband (I began to think I was being paranoid, given Jaycee's history); Jason wasn't sure if we should be worried or not. I sat on the concerns for a few months, not wanting to make something of nothing. Elijah's language development was on track, he was smart, and had a great memory. I used these positives to convince myself that problems with his motor skills were no big deal.

Finally, I decided to talk to his pediatrician. It's very weird to discuss concerns with a doctor, especially if you are the only one bringing it up. On one hand, I didn't want anything to be wrong with Elijah, yet I didn't want to look too focused or delusional over one little problem. The first time I brought it up, I was encouraged to keep Elijah from sitting in a "W" pattern on the floor and give him a little time. The doctor also encouraged me to have Elijah play at a table instead of on the floor in order to get him to sit with better posture.

I found the suggestions were easier said than done. After the conversation, I purchased a table and chair set to encourage Elijah to play while sitting on his bottom. Unfortunately, he preferred to sit on the floor and play. Every time I told Elijah to fix his legs from his "W" position, he would briefly take them out only to return his legs in that pattern again without him even realizing what he was doing. It was a full-time job to say, "Keep your legs in front."

The next time Elijah went to the doctor, I brought it up again. The doctor watched him walk, jump, and run. He agreed he should be seen by physical therapy to determine the issue. It was a happy and sad moment. I wouldn't have to wonder if a problem existed anymore, since someone would either confirm or deny it, however, I didn't really want him to need therapy.

I decided to take him for an outpatient therapy evaluation at a local hospital when he was around two-and-a-half-years old. I learned he sat like that because his core was weak. With that, he qualified for therapy, which aimed to improve his motor skills, strengthen his core muscles, and teach him better positioning. Elijah loved going to physical therapy. Unlike his sister who often refused many therapy exercises over the years, Elijah enjoyed having the attention and doing activities with a therapist. It was nice to take a child to therapy and not worry if he would be compliant or not.

Over the course of several weeks, Elijah made steady progress. By the time he was discharged, he was running. Granted, he was not running fast but he was running without falling. I was happy to see him make quick progress; I watched Jaycee complete therapy session after therapy session with very, very slow progress, despite all her hard work. It was nice seeing measurable improvement and it was motivating for both Elijah and me.

By the time Elijah was three, he was ready to attend pre-school and had been out of physical therapy for a little while. I was most interested in getting him in pre-school for social reasons, especially since his nonverbal sister rarely played with him. It made him extremely shy around other children and reluctant to join in with them, preferring to play by himself. His motor skills still had some small issues though; he could not pedal a bike, run fast, or perform harder tasks like hopping on one foot. Though he had some difficulties, he had many good abilities like memorizing information well. He knew all his letters and could sight read a few words before age three. Elijah grew up sitting next to me teaching Jaycee concepts, letters, numbers, and words and had absorbed much by being around Jaycee in those home-school sessions.

I was thrilled to learn our local pre-school had an opening for Elijah to start soon after he turned three. I knew it would be difficult for the both of us since I would miss him, but it was just a few hours each morning and not all day like when his sister attended. Elijah would have a hard time adjusting to school, but it would be the best thing for him in the long run. He was so shy! He rarely talked to his aunt, uncle, and grandma who cared for him while I worked, so his social skills were limited. At times, he seemed to have social anxiety, and I knew he needed to work this out in pre-school before kindergarten started.

Elijah reacted to school as I expected he would; he rarely talked to his teacher, kept to himself, and played near children but not with them. He slowly adjusted but the great thing was he enjoyed school, which surprised me. He liked to learn facts and have new experiences at school, which was exciting for him.

Halfway into the first year of pre-school, the teacher approached me about some concerns she had with him. Elijah was sitting in a "W" pattern on the floor at school and sat on his knees when in a chair. He still could not pedal a bike, his pencil grasp was light, and he struggled to copy shapes. Buttoning and zipping was something else that he could not do. Like me, she felt he was cognitively fine, but his motor skills were affecting him in school.

I soon found myself in a meeting to give consent for physical therapy and occupational therapy to evaluate Elijah, observe him in the classroom, and decide what types of support he needed, if any. I was fine with this evaluation since I saw him still struggling in those areas, too. As a therapist, I knew the sooner things were addressed, the better off he would be. Still, his scores would have to be low to qualify for services at the school. I figured that even with the issues, I was aware the possibility of him qualifying for services was slim. Boy, was I wrong!

A couple of months later, I was back at the pre-school to discuss my second child with this same group of people I had come to know well. I was nervous going into the meeting but expecting Elijah to be slightly delayed. He wasn't. In fact, it was the opposite.

Both therapists assessing his gross and fine motor skills found delays with Elijah. When his percentile ranks were read, my jaw dropped. I had no idea things were so bad. I suppose compared to Jaycee, Elijah's motor issues seemed minor. These reports helped me understand they weren't.

By: Evana Sandusky

Not only were his fine and gross motor skills delayed, but his overall tone was low also. He, like his sister, had hypotonia, though not as severe as Jaycee. His core muscles were extremely weak, which was affecting his ability to sit properly and, in turn, prevented him from writing letters or shapes properly.

While hearing the news of how Elijah performed, I had a thousand questions, but I only asked a few of them. If he is this delayed, why was his physical therapy in the hospital ever stopped? Why does he have hypotonia? Is there some underlying condition that I am oblivious to?

Really, I was shocked. I knew he had struggles, but I had no idea it was to the extent I was told. I let his good language and cognitive skills cloud my judgement. The team agreed his only issues were his motor skills. Still, having delays in both fine and gross motor, his official school diagnosis was developmental delay. Weekly physical and occupational therapy was started to help him develop.

After I signed the paperwork consenting to therapy services, I left the school meeting with an unexpected I.E.P. in my hand. When I got home, I looked over every word trying to make sense of what just happened. I read and re-read it, wondering why my son's muscles were so weak. I cried; I never imagined I would have two children receiving services. More than that, I cried because I was caught off guard completely by the test results. I wish I would have had some warning. I suppose the fact that we were having the meeting should have been some indication, but I was foolishly optimistic. The words *developmental delay* stung and showed I lacked an ability to gauge my own son's problems.

As time went on, I became fine with the idea that both of my children needed help. I was glad Elijah's teacher was brave enough to broach the subject with me. I was open to testing and willing to learn the results, whatever they may be because, in the end, all that mattered was giving my children the help they need to do their best. For some, that means specialized therapy.

Elijah made progress in therapy. His tone soon improved enough that he pedaled a tricycle and eventually a bicycle. By the time he entered kindergarten, he was able to write letters and keep up with classmates. Sometimes his letters were sloppy and huge, but he wrote them.

There were times when Elijah's motor delays were obvious to him and me. When he played tee ball, Jason and I marveled at how his muscle weakness impacted his ability to play. The bat used for tee ball seemed much too heavy for Elijah; he had to practice holding it up and swinging it before he could even think about hitting a ball. As he has gotten older, Elijah has come home from school remarking that his friends at school can run faster than him, which upsets and disappoints him that he is different athletically compared to the others in his class. I try to reassure him everyone has unique abilities and then I remind him of all the things he can do well. I try to help him understand that being first in sports isn't that important in life. These moments remind me how hard he must work to do things other children do naturally.

At the time of writing this, I still sit in a yearly meeting with Elijah's I.E.P. team. He has made good progress despite his muscle weakness. His delays probably aren't noticeable to most people now, which can be both a good and a bad thing. One day, I know Elijah will have a final I.E.P. meeting. Whether that day comes next year or in five years, it won't matter. I'll spend that special day reflecting on all he has accomplished and all the hard work he has put in over the years. I will also remember the lessons I have learned from receiving this unexpected badge.

Looking back, I don't know why I allowed myself to be so emotional over the I.E.P. Badges. My children needed help and thankfully there were programs to support them. These badges didn't carry the weight I thought they would when I first feared them years ago when Jaycee was born. For such a long time, these badges seemed like neon signs on my sash, but now I barely even think about them. My kids are who they are. They have needed some extra services to help them achieve what their peers do naturally but it's not that big of a deal. I just wish I would have realized that years ago.

CHAPTER 16:

THE WISH BADGE

Wish Badge: This badge is presented to the parent whose child has a dream come true from a wish granting charity. Though the wish granted is for the child, this badge symbolizes the mother's journey with her child. This badge is the symbol the mother has had an unusual parenting experience. This badge can be earned only once per child when the wish is granted.

Wish Badge Earned: 2015

I had been approached about determining if Jaycee would qualify for a Wish a few times prior to 2015. During her WPW scare and ablations, I considered starting the process, but I just couldn't do it. I didn't know if my child was "sick" enough. She did not have any one diagnosis that automatically qualified her for a wish, which meant her entire health history would have to be reviewed to decide if she was eligible. I had mixed feelings about this because if she didn't qualify, I would have felt bad for trying when so many kids need the Wish experience. If she did qualify, she would only get one wish; I wasn't sure if it was the right time to pursue it for her.

I decided to wait. If she would be eligible, I wanted Jaycee to be old enough to hopefully have some sort of say in what she would do. I also wanted her to be old enough to be able to remember it.

My mind began to change a few years later. In 2014, a social worker approached us about the idea of making a wish while Jaycee was in the ICU. At that point, Jaycee was doing her twice daily airway clearance to help her lung issues and she was taking several medications. She had been through some scary times in the ICU, and this one was no different. It was the first time we gave a Wish some serious thought. Jaycee's future no longer seemed guaranteed as a simple cold could do so much damage to her body she could end up in the ICU on respiratory support. With fear of the unknown future being my motivator, I decided it would be a good time to pursue this for Jaycee. She deserved some happiness, and this would surely bring her some.

The social worker offered to start the wish application process for us, so Jason and I consented. For one reason or another, we were discharged from the hospital without ever hearing back from the social worker. Once we got home, all my energy went into nursing Jaycee back to health. A few weeks later when things settled down, I decided to make the call to the Make-A-Wish Foundation myself.

During the call, they took down basic information about Jaycee, wanting to know all her diagnoses, surgeries, and current medications. They asked if any surgeries or appointments were upcoming and for the contact information for her pulmonary and cardiac doctors, who they would contact regarding the status of her health.

For some reason, I had strong emotions after I made the call. Again, I found myself crying in shock of what I had just done. I had heard about this organization helping children with life-threatening conditions and never imagined my child would ever be one of them. This call felt like an admission that my child's medical issues and health problems should not be minimalized. The call I placed was accepting something deeper in Jaycee's life, one I had not acknowledged before.

I was nervous in the weeks waiting to hear back regarding her eligibility. Then one sunny afternoon day when I was driving I received the phone call. Jaycee was eligible to receive a Wish

By: Evana Sandusky

based upon her lung conditions. I was happy for Jaycee. The remainder of the conversation focused on Jaycee's likes and dislikes, instead of her medical issues. I told them she loved the color green, Disney and Barney movies, and music. We were told to be thinking about possible Wishes for Jaycee and basically nothing was off limits as long as it was developmentally and medically appropriate.

After the news, Jason and I had to think of potential Wishes for Jaycee because she was essentially nonverbal, so we couldn't ask her what she wanted. She also didn't understand the idea of a Wish or could convey her deepest dreams with us. While Jaycee couldn't tell us what she wanted, we could keep her preferences in mind. We decided a trip would be the right Wish for her and would be something we normally wouldn't be able to offer her.

One thing we knew about Jaycee was she loved music and movies. Her collection of DVDs have been watched endlessly during her illnesses or daily vest therapy. Ultimately, these sparked our brainstorming. We were able to narrow some options down after talking to our local Wish volunteer who visited us at our home.

Due to her love of movies and characters, my husband and I decided on two possible trips. One option would be to California to visit Disneyland and a few other popular sites in the area while the other would be to Walt Disney World in Orlando, Florida and stay at Give Kids the World Village, which is a special resort exclusively for families of children on wish trips. We felt both would be great for Jaycee and she would enjoy either. Jason and I couldn't decide as we weighed the pros and cons for each. California would be a longer flight, which was a negative. We had been to Orlando once, but this would be a completely different experience as a Wish family. Elijah wanted California because he wanted to see the Cars area at Disneyland and, honestly, I was a little partial to California, too.

Nevertheless, we wanted the choice to be Jaycee's, so I came up with a way to let her decide. Since she is accustomed to communicating in pictures, I used pictures to help her make a choice. I made a poster of the things we would do in California. There was a picture of an airplane, Princess Sofia, Disneyland, a dolphin, and Lightning McQueen. For Florida, there were pictures of an airplane, Barney the dinosaur, Santa Claus (because he would be at Give Kids the World), ice cream, Princess Sofia, and a picture of the Magic Kingdom. I talked to Jaycee about every picture on each page. Then I asked her, "Which one do you like?"

I kept a tally of her responses. But, after a while I didn't need a tally sheet. She clearly wanted to go to Florida, which upset Elijah.

After that, the wheels were set into motion. Jaycee was going to receive a trip to Orlando to visit the theme parks and stay at Give Kids the World Village. As a bonus, Jaycee was going to meet Barney the Dinosaur, which was a favorite of hers at the time. We chose to go in February when temperatures were not too hot and when the crowds were lower. Jaycee, in general, was usually healthy around that time of the year too, which was another positive aspect.

The date for the departure for our trip became circled on our calendar and excitement built. There are so many dates in a calendar year for us, but most of them have to do with doctors' appointments and tests. It was so amazing to have a happy date to look forward to on the calendar.

During this waiting period, we had several talks with the children to prepare them for what was going to happen. Neither of them had ever been on an airplane before, so it was going to be a new experience for them. I read airplane stories and discussed the security screening process with the children, so they wouldn't be scared. In the meantime, I researched how I would travel with Jaycee's BiPAP, vest airway clearance machine, nebulizer, and liquid medications.

Explaining to Elijah why Jaycee was receiving the Wish was important. As a 5-year-old, he questioned why he wasn't going to get a Wish someday, so I needed to clear this up for him. Elijah has always visited Jaycee when she was in the hospital and heard us say we couldn't do things from time to time because of Jaycee's health. With that knowledge, I was able to help him understand. He was a little jealous of his sister, but that is understandable. For a child, he coveted picking a special activity, too. I tried to remind him he was going on Jaycee's trip, so he would benefit from it as well.

Before the trip, I wanted to prepare Elijah for the other children he might see at the Give Kids the World Village. With other experiences in the hospital, Elijah had heard of things like cancer, breathing machines, and wheelchairs and they were part of his vocabulary, yet he didn't have a full grasp of them. I started telling him how the other children in the village all were there because someone was sick or had health problems like his sister. I explained how some of the children might be in wheelchairs, some might not have hair, and some might just look different than us. He seemed unphased by the information and excited to see the village.

After a few months, the much-anticipated day for the trip through the Make-A-Wish Foundation came. Being two hours from the airport and having to fly out early in the morning, we stayed in a hotel closer to the airport the night before to make things easier. We were all so excited about starting this special trip! At 6:30 in the morning, a limousine arrived to take us to the airport. Elijah loved the limo ride, but Jaycee was confused by it at first; she did not like having a chauffeur and wondered why he was touching our luggage.

Off to the airport we went riding in style like we were celebrities. The airport security was our first big test with Jaycee. Of course, Jaycee's vest therapy machine, nebulizer, liquid medication, and BiPAP machine were all flagged by security for an additional screening, but we had anticipated it. Jaycee did well listening as we made our way through security and waited for our flight. Fortunately, the airport was not too busy that day. I don't think we looked too confused making our way through the airport either.

After the first hurdle of security, I became nervous about Jaycee flying in an airplane. I never know how Jaycee will react to a new situation. If she didn't like it, it was going to be a long, stressful flight. That wasn't an issue though because Jaycee loved it. Both kids did great actually! If anyone was tense during the flight, it was me. I seemed to be the only person looking around and grabbing the armrests of the seats when we flew through mild turbulence.

We arrived at the Orlando International airport and looked for the greeters waiting for us from Give Kids the World Village. They were easy to spot, and they guided us through picking up our bags and getting our rental car. We would have been lost without them! We are not big-time city people or travelers, so this was all new for us! The airport appeared to have more people in it than our entire little town we lived in.

Give Kids the World village was about a 40-minute drive. I was looking forward to having Jaycee experience all the fun at the village and to see this amazing place for myself. From the moment we arrived, we were greeted with happy, smiling people who seemed to love being there. We checked in and were shown the little villa that would be ours for the rest of the week. It was truly amazing. Having our own house to stay in versus a hotel room was so wonderful given all the things we needed for Jaycee. The kids loved sharing a bedroom and having their own bathroom, too. There was also WIFI, a kitchen, a living room, and a washer/dryer. Snacks were waiting for us as well as gifts for the kids. It was clear the village took pride in having nice accommodations for the families.

After we settled in, I attended the village orientation to learn about everything we would have access to and all the amenities available during our stay. Besides free theme park tickets, almost every theme park gave us a special pass that allowed us to go to the head of the lines. Skipping the long lines to meet characters or get on a ride meant Jaycee would not wear down so quickly. That ended up being the best perk of the trip for us! We were also able to eat meals at the village for free. We could also eat ice cream free anytime the ice cream shop was open! Mini-golf, swimming, carousel rides, an arcade, and more were all on the grounds as well. All this village had to offer families was completely unbelievable.

After I finished orientation, we took the rest of the afternoon and evening to explore the village. The carousel was an immediate hit with our family. We checked out the arcade, watched an amazing model train display, and drove some toy boats. We made special pillows in the castle, got ice cream, and swam in their heated pool. Jaycee loves to swim, so that was her favorite! We found out that we needed to be in a heated pool in Florida in February.

The most common phrase our family used through the first few hours at the village was, "Wow! Look at this!"

At the end of the first day, I realized the trip was the right decision for Jaycee. Prior to the trip, the only thing that concerned me about the village was it would mean being surrounded by other children with health conditions. I thought it might be depressing to see so many children in poor health. I wondered if it was going to be the happy place it claimed to be with so many families there in a multitude of health battles. After just a few hours, it was clear my concerns were invalid. The

By: Evana Sandusky

many volunteers from around the world were happy to serve, the paid staff were happy, and the other families were all happy. It was kind of amazing to see so many blissful people in one place. I, too, was joyful as I went to bed that first night. Jaycee had a full week of adventure ahead of her. I could not wait!

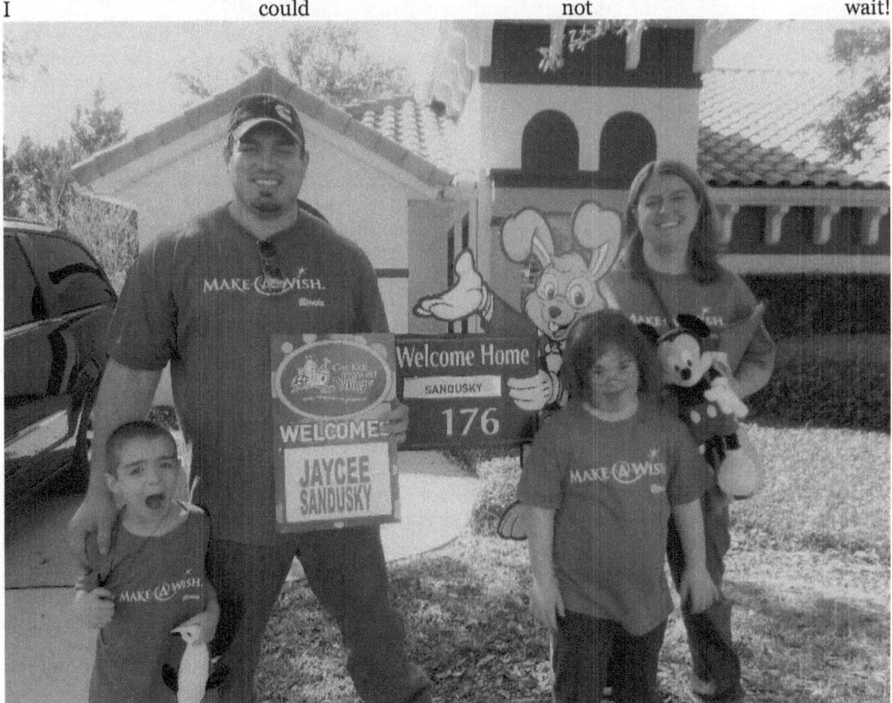

Our first full day in Florida for our trip was busy. We knew this was a once in a lifetime experience, so we were determined to do as much as possible, especially since Jaycee was in good health at the time. Each morning, there were different characters available to meet and greet at the village. We were able to see Mickey, Goofy, and Pluto. Jaycee was in heaven already meeting her favorite characters and we hadn't left the Village yet!

After breakfast, we drove to the Animal Kingdom. Having had a Disney vacation before, we knew what we wanted to see and do at each Disney theme park. Jaycee loves certain animals, so we made sure we saw those early in the day when she was full of energy. Then the rain started. Oh, Florida and its sudden rain showers! We took cover in the Rainforest Café, where we learned Jaycee would receive a complementary meal for being a Wish child.

After our big lunch, we headed to Hollywood Studios. We had many characters and shows on the agenda. The boys headed to some "manly" shows while Jaycee and I went to watch the *Frozen* show, which she absolutely loved. After the show, Jaycee was invited to meet the *Frozen* characters privately. She was in heaven again being able to touch and talk to Anna and Elsa. The characters were so friendly and spent some precious time with Jaycee. It was amazing!

While the whole family walked through Hollywood Studios, one of the green army men (from *Toy Story*) spotted my shirt that indicated we were on a Wish trip. He literally waved us down and gestured to follow him. I didn't know what we were doing since the army men do not speak, but we did as commanded. We were soon surrounded by two more army men who danced with Jaycee and acted silly. Then we were taken to a room to meet Buzz and Woody. The picture we got was awesome! The army men, Buzz, and Woody surrounded Jaycee and our family. I felt like we were celebrities being given the royal treatment!

As we left Hollywood Studios, Jaycee signed to her dad about meeting Elsa and Anna and how she and I watched the *Beauty and the Beast* show. Elijah told us about seeing some car shows and other intriguing activities. When we returned to the village, the children were surprised to see gifts sitting on the table for them. This happened every day! The gifts ranged from board games to jewelry to stuffed animals and toys. It was an added thrill for them every day to see what was waiting for them inside. After they tore through their gifts, we still had ice cream to eat and a few rides to go on before going to bed. We never once said we were bored during our stay. Our main complaint was there was too much to do and not enough hours in the day to do it.

The next day, I woke up extremely excited because it was Jaycee's day to meet Barney the dinosaur. Jaycee had a huge smile on her face as the day started at the village with a meet and greet with Dora the Explorer. Then it was on to Universal Studios for the day!

Universal Studios is a huge place that we tried to cram into one day. Jaycee was brave enough to do many rides that I thought were questionable for her age like the Spiderman and Transformers rides. We took in as much of the park as we could before our arranged time to meet Barney.

Jaycee got excited when she saw the Barney signs and décor outside of the Barney Theater. She knew exactly who we were going to see as she signed her own sign for "Barney." Since Jaycee was Barney's special guest for his live show, we were given a front row seat to watch him. My husband and I spent the entire production watching Jaycee watch the show. Her eyes lit up when Baby Bop, BJ, and Barney made their entrances. She smiled, danced, and giggled through the show. It was incredible seeing her so happy. How I wished she could talk in those moments. I would have loved to know exactly what she was thinking and feeling during the show. Obviously, she was ecstatic, but I wonder how amazed she felt to see Barney right in front of her. I never wanted that show to end! I was probably the only parent thinking that in the audience at the time.

After the show, Jaycee was invited to meet Barney one-on-one. She hugged Barney and looked at him with such adoration. We made sure this visit with Barney was well documented with photos. Seeing as Barney was "resting his voice" between shows, he and Jaycee communicated without words. They danced and held hands. They took a walk together around his theatre. Barney did not rush through this meeting; he gave my sweet Jaycee several precious minutes. I was not sure what to expect from this meet and greet with Barney, but it exceeded all my expectations. Jaycee was elated. What more could I ask for? Barney led Jaycee to a play area and then discreetly walked away. Jaycee was distracted, so the parting from Barney was smooth and easy. That Barney sure knew how to handle children!

After the Barney visit, we spent the next several hours seeing the rest of Universal. Jaycee was in character paradise meeting multiple characters ranging from Captain America to the Grinch. Of course, my son loved the superheroes at Universal; it was one of the highlights of the trip for him that otherwise involved so many princesses.

When the kids were meeting Captain America, he asked Elijah who his favorite superhero was for which Elijah responded, "Spiderman!" Captain America told him where to go to meet him and gave him a big smile. That Captain America is such a classy guy. A few years later, Captain America would become Elijah's favorite hero though, so hopefully Captain America wasn't crushed that day.

As much as we loved Universal, we wanted to be back at the village for the big event of the night, Mayor Clayton's birthday party. Mayor Clayton and his wife are two bunny characters (adults in costumes) who live at the village. Sometimes, you can see the bunnies literally driving around the village in a car, which was just as exciting for the adults as it was the children. There was going to be dancing for the party, which was a favorite activity for Jaycee. The kids made cards for the bunny and presented them to him. There were party games and food. It was fun and sweet time.

We left the festivities with the Mayor Clayton to do some other things going on around the village. The boys went fishing at the village pond while the girls hit the beauty salon. Jaycee got her nails painted green since it's her favorite color. She sat so well for her salon treatment, it surprised me.

After a busy day, we got the kids ready for bed, but we had one more surprise. We had scheduled a bedtime tuck-in for the kids with the Mayor. We could schedule one tuck-in from

By: Evana Sandusky

either the Mayor or his wife as an added activity at the village. The kids were happy to see the large rabbit in their room. Jaycee got so excited, she started jumping on her bed, which made Elijah jump on his bed. Mayor Clayton covered his eyes with his paws and shook his head in disbelief. He gestured for the kids to settle down and they complied. After the bunny covered them up and waved goodnight, he left our villa.

The day was simply magical. I was excited Jaycee got to meet Barney and went to bed feeling so grateful for the experience. I loved that Jaycee had this wonderful trip to make happy memories. I hadn't felt this joyful in years. I know Jaycee must have had a similar feeling.

On Wednesday, we decided to pace ourselves, so we could enjoy fireworks at Epcot that night. Jaycee's stamina was not the greatest, and we had pushed her hard already. We decided to have an easy morning at the village instead. First, we took advantage of the free horse rides available. Prior to this, Jaycee had a few pony rides at fairs but hadn't had a recent experience with a horse. To our surprise, Jaycee was in love with the horses! When her turn was over, she signed, "My turn, horse!" She even tried to say the word horse for the first time ever. Jaycee had a few extra rides on the horse before we left the area. We had no idea she would love horse rides so much. That was the beauty of this experience; we got to try so many new things with Jaycee and learn more about her preferences.

After the horse rides, we tried out the miniature golf course on the village grounds. The kids had never golfed before, so we thought this would be a good place to give it a try. What can I say? The kids had a really great time, but they never golfed. Jaycee hit any ball she found whether it was hers or not; Elijah kept using his club backwards. When Jaycee got tired of hitting her ball, she would throw it in the hole or wander off. I found the whole thing humorous. Jason found it frustrating as he did his best to teach a game he enjoyed to the kids. We were certainly glad this first-time experience was free because it was a complete and utter disaster if actual golfing was the goal.

We gave up on golf before finishing all the holes and decided we should have some ice cream at the village. It was 10:30 in the morning, and I felt like a rebel encouraging my children to choose an ice cream snack so early in the day. The kids could get whatever ice cream treat they wanted, and they were so happy. The normal rules don't apply on a Wish trip!

We made a quick stop at Downtown Disney for some shopping before heading into Epcot for the rest of the day. Elijah wanted to go to the Lego store and desired to purchase as much as possible on a $30 budget. Meanwhile, Jaycee had big plans to get a princess dress complete with shoes and accessories. After she looked through every available dress, she finally settled on a Cinderella dress. I loved every minute of shopping with her. I felt like just an ordinary mom with her daughter.

At Epcot, we rode a few rides before getting in line to see all the princesses. Jaycee enjoyed seeing Belle, Sleeping Beauty, Jasmine, and Snow White. Elijah was, as you can imagine, bored! He was happier when we met Goofy and Mickey later, since no tiaras were involved.

We easily managed to keep busy until it was time for the fireworks. I can't stress how uncharacteristic it was for me to stay out late with my children for something like evening fireworks. Due to Jaycee's nightly 50 minutes of medications and vest therapy treatments, I generally do not like to stay out late. The dread of having to do that medication run when Jaycee is tired and grumpy late at night is enough for me to say no to anything that occurs after 7 p.m. My husband convinced me to be more flexible and not let her medical needs dictate our fun.

The fireworks and show were amazing. Jaycee loved it, which made it worthwhile. I was glad I listened to Jason. We had a late night of doing all her medications after we arrived back at the village, but it was worth the extra work.

The next day we woke up to chilly temperatures, wind, and rain in the forecast. After a stop in the village to see Belle again, we decided to look for an indoor activity available. We opted to go to the Kennedy Space Center at Cape Canaveral since it was a short drive away. Before the rain started, we explored all the outdoor rockets. Elijah marveled at their size and peppered us with questions we couldn't answer. We decided to try an IMAX movie available at the center. This was a new experience for the children, so I was concerned about Jaycee during the movie. I could not get her to try on the 3D glasses, so the entire movie must have been blurry to her. I wondered what she was thinking as the movie played. However, she sat well though and we managed to make it through the whole thing.

The weather started to get awful while we were there, so we went on the bus tour to see the launch areas. Jason and I were enjoying the space center, but our kids were not. It was geared more towards adults for sure. After hearing the children complain they were freezing in the windy, rainy weather, we decided to leave without seeing a big part of the space center. I was glad we went to see it, but it just wasn't a good fit with our children.

We arrived back at the village in time for dinner. Thursday night's activity was Christmas at the village (even though it was February), which meant Santa, Christmas carols, and Christmas decorations. It was a joyful, happy evening. Jaycee debuted her new Cinderella princess dress, which drew comments from all the volunteers at the village. She loved being a princess when she met Santa. After some pictures with Santa, we were escorted in to a room filled with toys. The kids were directed to shelves stacked with toys for their age and were able to select one toy to take home and keep. As I had several times before in the week, I stood amazed by everything this village had to offer for our family and all the other families on Wish trips. It was absolutely astounding to think of all the donations, volunteers, and materials needed to keep this place going day after day for years. It's a magical place of its own with a true display of generosity found nowhere else I had been in this country.

We woke up to better weather on Friday, thankfully. We headed to the Magic Kingdom early to be there when the gates opened, since it was one of our favorite theme parks. Jaycee was thrilled to meet Cinderella, Elsa, Anna, and other friends. It didn't matter if she had already met a character before, she wanted to meet her again. She let me meet a few of the characters with her, but she wasn't too happy about her mom invading her special time. She would stomp her feet and tell me I was making her mad. I guess she knew this special trip was all for her.

Our favorite ride at the Magic Kingdom was the Seven Dwarfs Mine Train. We rode it as a family together repeatedly. When the ride attendant heard my son say we should ride it again, he immediately escorted us back to the front of the line. Wow! We felt so special! But, we only did that once since there were many people waiting in line. Disney parks really go above and beyond to make the kids on Wish trips feel special.

We ended up staying at the park until 7 pm. Of course, by that time in the trip, Jaycee was always using her wheelchair instead of walking or standing in line. She was exhausted but able to keep going with the wheelchair, which saved her energy. Jason and I got a workout pushing her everywhere all week.

We arrived back at the village too late to eat the family buffet dinner available every night, but we were able to use their pizza delivery service. While we waited on the pizza, Jaycee did her evening medicine regime. It was late and cold, but I was determined to take Jaycee for one more swim. We had so many things to do during our week at the village that we had only swam once. Thank God the pool was heated because the air was cold. I was somewhat worried about Jaycee being wet in cold air with her lung problems. If we were back home, I never would have considered this activity due to the risks. Still, I tried to let her have fun and not stress about a potential health risk. We were the only two people swimming in the pool, so we had the large pool all to ourselves. Everyone else probably knew it was way too cold to swim. Elijah and Jason enjoyed cold ice cream while Jaycee and I were just cold.

I felt a little sad after the swim, as it was our last night at the village. We had a wonderful time, and I wasn't ready to leave the place where we were treated with such love and my children were so jubilant. I was so glad Jaycee chose this for her Wish. She fit right in at the village; she wasn't an anomaly there.

Jaycee can walk, but not as much as the trip required. She wasn't the only child using a wheelchair though. Not only that, people instinctively knew to open doors for us if they saw us coming, and everything was accessible (even the pool), which was so wonderful for all the other families as well. If I gave Jaycee a syringe of medicine at dinner, no one stared. When I mixed things into her drinks, no one seemed interested. We didn't stick out like we would in other public places. I felt like I belonged there among all the other strangers who endured hardships like us.

While we only got to know a few other families there at the village, we felt a connection to almost everyone we met. We understood that behind the smiling parents watching their child play,

By: Evana Sandusky

swim, or meet a beloved character, there was a story and a reason that brought them to the village. It was that common ground that spurred the love and kindness felt everywhere we went in the village.

One night, I said to Elijah, "Isn't the village nice? And there are other children in wheelchairs just like your sister uses."

His response was, "There were? I didn't notice."

Elijah is one of a kind!

The next morning, we had to pack up our belongings and check out of the village. We all felt grateful to experience such a wonderful place but sad to leave so soon. Each Wish child is allowed one week; as our time was up, another child and his or her family would soon be taking our place. After breakfast, we let Jaycee enjoy the horse rides that were back at the village. She still loved them and wanted to stay with them as long as she could. Jaycee took more than one ride on the horses again and smiled the entire time.

Our next stop that morning was the Castle of Miracles at the village to find Jaycee's star. Every Wish child that has been to the village has a star in the castle. Yes, there are thousands of stars. It's overwhelming to see each of them knowing they represent a child in a health battle. It's even harder to think that some of the stars are from children who lost their fight on Earth.

Earlier in the week, Jaycee had doodled on a golden star and then sent it off to the "star fairy," who would place the star somewhere in the castle. The star fairy delivered a letter to us a day or so later detailing the location of Jaycee's star in the castle. With the help of a volunteer, we were able to see where Jaycee's star would be forever. It was located too high to see the exact place it was, but they had pictures available for us. It was a touching moment that I emotionally didn't want to linger in. It was one of those times in life that was bittersweet. I was happy Jaycee had a star and experienced the village and saddened by what she and so many children had lived through to get there. I may have cried a little bit as we pulled away from the village that day. Our family was so blessed and touched by the week we had there, but our trip was not over yet.

The last official theme park on our Wish trip was Sea World. There we were again given front of the line access at rides, special seating at the shows, and a free wheelchair rental. We were excited to attend Jack Hannah's animal show, but Jaycee was not. It was a dark theater, so she immediately sunk to the floor until she felt safe enough to sit in her seat. That moment occurred when the show was pretty much over. To our surprise, Jaycee really loved the dolphin and killer whale shows; she danced and cheered throughout them. The outdoor and well-lit amphitheater was a better fit for her I suppose. It was again wonderful to experience something new and for her to love it so much.

The Sea World staff was kind and accommodating to us. The other people though, that's another story. Everyone wants to see the marine life and only focus on their child being able to catch a glimpse of a fascinating creature in an exhibit. Getting Jaycee in her wheelchair close enough to see the exhibits was next to impossible. By that time in the trip, she was exhausted and really didn't want to stand or walk any more than absolutely needed. We were tired from the exhausting schedule we put ourselves through, so we could only imagine how Jaycee felt. She was not able to stand and walk around to see any of the exhibits that required you to step up for a closer look. Jason and I would wait patiently behind people taking in their view from the rail; as soon as they walked away, we could not push Jaycee the two feet forward to be at the rail fast enough. There was always someone who filed into the spot that we were desperately trying to bring our daughter. After being in parks all week and everyone in our family worn down, we quickly ran out of energy to fight the crowds for a glimpse of whatever it was we were not able to see.

Unfortunately, we ended up leaving Sea World early without seeing half of it. Maybe we'll get another chance to go when Jaycee is able to walk and fight for a spot to see things for herself. I hated that we couldn't make the most of the day at Sea World, but our mental happiness was more important at that point.

When we left Sea World, we were officially vacationing on our own. Before our trip, I had researched the experiences of other families who shared their stories online. Most people recommended staying for a few more days to decompress and relax before flying home, since the actual Wish trip was jam-packed with excitement. We decided to follow their advice and drove to the Cape Canaveral area. We checked into a resort where we would spend the last leg of our trip.

While we were vacationing on our own at Cape Canaveral, all our meals and other expenses were our responsibility. No one was aware we were on a Wish trip now unless we told them, which rarely ever happened.

We stayed on a resort near Cocoa Beach, so we could be near the ocean. Our room at the resort was lovely but it felt small after the accommodations at the village. Our luggage and Jaycee's equipment filled every space of our room, which is the norm in any hotel we stay. We were back to normal life as regular people on vacation. We enjoyed a small water park the resort had to offer but missed the heated water at the village. Jaycee finally got to swim during the day when it wasn't freezing, which was nice.

We were slammed back into reality at the resort's indoor playground that was full of healthy, typical kids. It was the usual encounter and comments of children asking if Jaycee could talk and why not. Most of the questions were directed to her brother as he introduced his sister to the new children. We were sheltered at the village among people like us and I found myself, once again, that mom seeing children notice Jaycee's differences and trying to decide if it's worth my energy on vacation to step in or ignore them. I let Elijah handle it on his own, as he was doing a great job.

"She's my sister. Her name is Jaycee. She can't talk," he told the enthusiastic listeners. Well done, son!

I was eager to leave the resort area and have the kids experience the ocean for the first time. I didn't know how Jaycee would react to the beach. She doesn't like sand in general, but we had never experienced the soft sand found only on an ocean beach. There's nothing like it in Illinois! Me, being the planner, had already discussed with Jason how we would each get back to the room if Jaycee was too overstimulated and needed to get off the beach quickly. We never had to use the plan though. She absolutely loved the beach! The water wasn't warm enough to swim in, but we enjoyed the few inches we dipped into and playing in the sand. Elijah loved collecting sea shells and building sand castles. Jaycee liked laying on the beach. She was very content to watch the waves and feel the sand in her toes. I like any place she's laying down instead of running off from me. I was very surprised how calming the beach was for her.

I found the beach extremely relaxing as well. It was probably the most relaxed I had felt in years laying in that soft sand and hearing the gentle roar of the ocean waves. Before the trip, I wasn't sure if I could unwind enough to enjoy the beach. I'm not really a sit-outside-and-enjoy-nature person, but this was so peaceful. Jaycee and I laid on our towels right next to each other, held hands, and took in the view. For a moment, the world seemed to disappear around us. We were just a mother and daughter without a care in the world. It felt great.

We couldn't just lay around on the beach all day, and Jason and I did not want to pass up the opportunities to experience more unique activities. We decided to take a popular tourist air boat ride to see alligators in the area. There again, I was reluctant to do this activity because I was unsure of how Jaycee would react to an air boat, but Jason once again encouraged me. I had visions of Jaycee trying to jump off the boat because of the wind and noise frightening her. Fortunately, Jason was right again! Both kids loved it and smiled as we spotted gators from a safe distance. We did less adventurous activities too, such as shopping and trying new restaurants. I always know those are safe activities for Jaycee.

Before we knew it, it was time to pack up and leave the magic and excitement of Florida. Not one of us wanted to leave. When Elijah voiced his displeasure of the trip ending, we reminded him that there are other children like his sister who need to make these trips too. Still, I wanted to sit and cry too! *I didn't want any of it to end.* We were having such a great time. All the stress from years of caring for Jaycee was kept at a distance on this trip. I didn't want that feeling back. I wasn't ready to go home and face future doctor appointments, pharmacy pick-ups, and all the rest of it.

We will forever be grateful to the Make-A-Wish Foundation, the Wish volunteers (especially Alison and Gwen), Give Kids the World Village, and the all the companies who continue to come together to make these trips so exceptional for families like ours. Jason and I both feel we will never have another trip as special and unique as that one; we felt privileged to share this incredible experience with Jaycee.

The trip has continued to bring us joy years later. We love sharing about our adventures in Florida with others and looking at our keepsakes we brought home. Because Jaycee's speech is limited, I really wanted to make sure she had reminders of the trip around her, so she could

By: Evana Sandusky

communicate about the trip in some way. I made a few scrapbooks and picture albums, trying to capture every memory for Jaycee. We had many pictures printed off to hang throughout our house as well. I made a video with all the pictures we collected too, since Jaycee loves movies. The Wish trip was well documented, so Jaycee should always remember it. We won't ever let her forget though.

The Wish Badge became pinned to my sash representing the happy, once-in-a-lifetime experience we had. What I thought might be a depressing badge at first became one of the cheeriest and freeing moments as a mother in my life.

CHAPTER 17:

THE CHILD BAPTISM BADGE

> *Child Baptism Badge: This badge is awarded to the Christian mom for each of her children who are water baptized. This badge represents the faith the mother has passed on to her child.*

Child Baptism Badge Earned: October 19, 2014

Being in the Christian faith, the sacrament of baptism is extremely important to me. There are several different ideas on when baptism should occur within our faith. For me, I believe a person is baptized after he or she has decided to become a follower of Jesus. Salvation first, then baptism has been my church experience, but this may differ for others.

I sat through many water baptisms at church after my daughter was born with a bit of jealousy and sadness. While I was happy for the children I witnessed being baptized at our church, I couldn't help but think of my daughter.

Will Jaycee live long enough to be baptized? Will Jaycee understand the concept of baptism in order to be baptized?

Every baptism I watched when Jaycee was younger caused me to pray that I would one day see my daughter baptized. It was my heart's desire like any other mother in our faith.

After Jaycee's scary ICU stay in 2013, I had a desire to see Jaycee baptized. It was a thought that came to me occasionally when she had fully recovered and was back home. At first, I didn't even know what to think about getting Jaycee baptized. It felt like it was my decision and not my daughter's, so that seemed contradictory to my beliefs regarding baptism.

Due to Jaycee's limited comprehension and minimal verbal speech, it was impossible to really know if she understood concepts like Jesus, God, salvation, and baptism. There wasn't a way for her to really receive salvation under those circumstances either, since she could not say a typical prayer of salvation. It didn't seem fair that Jaycee couldn't technically do the required steps and may never be able to fulfill them. After all, we were raising her in the faith, and we considered her a part of the church body—didn't that count for something? Even if I was the one encouraging the baptism, was it wrong? If Jaycee never had the ability to initiate it on her own, then maybe I needed to lead her through the process like I do as a parent in so many areas. I spent a great deal of time meditating on these things and trying to figure out what I really believed.

Like any person with a wild idea, I sat on it, I meditated on it, and I wondered how it would happen. I finally broached the subject with my husband. He had the same concerns as me and neither of us had a good answer.

Did you ever have an exciting idea that just fizzled away over time? Initially, I was eager about this idea of baptism for Jaycee even though I had reservations. I let the doubt and questions fill my mind. Soon, the excitement and wonderment of this possibility seemed to just slowly fade.

Then, out of the blue months later, I was sitting in church when a thought came to mind. *You never had Jaycee baptized. Oh yes! I did mean to have that done.*

The timing of that reminder could only have been from God because a few days later there was a reason for urgency to get the baptism completed. Jaycee went back in the ICU in July 2014, and it was a call to action for me. She was struggling to breath on the BiPAP machine and life was scary

By: Evana Sandusky

again. Jason and I looked totally defeated when the team of doctors prepared us for the possibility of her going on the ventilator again. Thankfully, things did not get to that point, but it was a wake-up call for me. Time was not a guarantee with Jaycee.

I looked at Jason across Jaycee's room and said, "If she makes it out of here alive, we are getting her baptized." He wholeheartedly agreed.

Once home, we had more talks about Jaycee, disability, and baptism. Jason's main concern was if her understanding improved one day to the point she could somehow verbalize her salvation and desire to be baptized what would happen as it would be done already. I reminded him that many people in the church are baptized as young children who then as adults choose to be re-baptized as a rededication to God. That situation hasn't been uncommon in churches we have attended. I saw Jaycee as no different. If she chose to do it again later, that could be her choice. If that chance never occurred or her health declined, then she was covered until then. Our conversations had led us to one conclusion—baptize Jaycee.

Once life settled down, I sat down and typed a very long email to our pastor. I didn't want to catch him off guard before or after a service with this idea. I wanted him to read it without pressure of giving an immediate answer. I told him that Jaycee being water baptized had been a desire of ours for a while, but I had been reluctant to do anything with the desire. I didn't want to have her baptized just because I was afraid she was going to die; I wanted to make sure my motives were from God and not from fear. I explained how I could not say for sure if Jaycee was "saved" due to her delays, I remarked that she loves church, worshipping along to songs, and knows how to pray in her own way. I hit send on that novel of an email and waited anxiously for a reply.

In the meantime, I told my parents, who also attend our church, about the situation. They thought it was a wonderful idea and supported the notion, especially given Jaycee's medical issues. They, like us, felt she should not be denied to perform a sacrament of our faith due to the technicality that she can't verbalize her thoughts about God. I was happy to have support because I was unsure of how people would react to this (for what I felt was an) unprecedented event.

I was determined to have her baptized in some way, no matter the outcome of the email. I started brainstorming other possible ministers we could use that were connected to Jaycee and her story if our pastor did not agree to do it. I thought of people with hot tubs or swimming pools that we may be able to contact to use to do the baptism if a church wasn't an option.

Finally, one day, I received a reply. Pastor Chad had prayed about this request. He agreed to have Jaycee baptized, replying he didn't have a strong conviction either way but was open to the idea if we were feeling led to do it.

After writing back and forth, we agreed on the terms and conditions of the baptism. Because we were not sure how Jaycee would react during the baptism, we decided to do it privately after service was over. This would give her extra time to get in and out of the baptistery. It would also allow all the family to surround her in the baptistery, which would help her feel more at ease. I liked the idea of a semi-private baptism. If someone had concerns about the legitimacy of Jaycee's act, I would be spared the questions. I found my peace on the subject through prayer, so I didn't really want the opinions of a bystander who probably wasn't fully aware of our situation anyway. Pastor Chad asked me if Jaycee had a fear of water and other things that may impede the process. We worked them out, and the date was set.

I had two big jobs after that. First, I had to invite friends and family to witness it, which meant I had to tell them about my radical idea. People were very kind and supportive. If someone thought it was a strange idea, no one told me. The second task I had was to prepare Jaycee for the big day. That took intentional effort.

I wanted Jaycee to understand what she was doing. Any child or person who does this religious act needs to understand the reason behind it; Jaycee was no different. A few weeks before the big day, I started preparing her. I found many YouTube videos that showed baptisms in all sorts of water receptacles. We even watched the baptism of Jesus from a movie. We read stories in her children's Bible about baptism, but the biggest thing I did to help her was writing my own little book on the subject just for her. It was a simple book that I knew she could understand and included my own poorly drawn illustrations.

Jaycee seemed responsive throughout all of this. As the date got closer, we told her about her big day at church and named everyone who would be there to see her. We told her she would, "Go down and right back up." This was the simple phrase I chose to remind her of the quickness of the event. A few days before the baptism, I started practicing in the bathtub with her. I never took her under the water, since she would only need to do that once for the real act. I did lean her back to wet her hair though. Through the trial runs, Jaycee was happy and wanted to practice more than once.

By the time the baptismal date arrived, I felt Jaycee was ready. After the regular Sunday service ended, many of our family and friends crowded on stage surrounding the baptistery. Jaycee entered the water going down the steps all by herself. She smiled as she looked at everyone. It didn't hurt that she likes being the center of attention. Pastor Chad said a few words and then reminded Jaycee that she would go down and right back up.

That's exactly what happened. She went down in the water and back up. She came out of the water smiling and happy. Jaycee was not at all scared by any of it, which I hope was because of my preparation. Jaycee was baptized—she did it!

Since that day, Jaycee has happily looked at the pictures and talked about her "swim" at church. Soon after, she took her first communion at church. She worked to get every drop of juice out of the tiny communion cup. If she could talk, I am sure she would question someone on the portion size of the juice and cracker.

With her baptism complete, my faith had successfully been passed on to Jaycee, but of course teaching her about God continued. I feel at peace with our decision and smile when I look down at the Child Baptism Badge.

While her baptism didn't go the normal route, it felt right to us. It also made me reflect upon the accommodations that need to be considered in the church for those with disabilities. We might be denying someone in the church an experience he or she is entitled to based upon a technicality that we feel is necessary but may be unrealistic.

Clearly, God has worked in Jaycee's life. There have been many times when her health events could have ended differently. The baptism was another way to acknowledge everything God had done for Jaycee. She was and is a child of God, even if she can't say it herself.

By: Evana Sandusky

EPILOGUE

I hope you have enjoyed reading the stories and experiences I have had while earning my badges of motherhood. All these stories are true, although at times they must sound unbelievable. When I was writing this book and thought back on events and experiences we have had, even I cannot believe the things my family has lived through. I feel blessed to be a mother and am grateful that Jaycee has lived through every health scare for the past twelve years and counting.

The lives of a mother and her children become intertwined and connected so much that one's life experience touches and affects the others. This book shared my perspective as a mother in many situations and events. That being said, I am fully aware that Jaycee was and is the one enduring the surgeries, living with chronic health conditions, and experiencing pains and fears I can't imagine. I never want to make her life experiences all about me. Yet, I have been right beside Jaycee for her entire life. I hope I have simply shared what my role as a mother was during some of those health scares and hospital admissions. I wish that one day Jaycee can be verbal enough to tell her side of these stories because she would have her own perspective on these same events.

Even though motherhood brought me experiences that I never anticipated, I enjoy and love my children. Their lives are valuable and God-given. Down syndrome and all the other diagnoses that came along for Jaycee, and even Elijah, have changed aspects of my life, but my life is good. My child's life is good. I only regret letting the fear of the diagnoses steal so much of my joy when they were given. Thankfully, I have grown as a person and a mother.

If you are raising a child with developmental and/or medical needs, I hope this book has given you some encouragement and helped you realize you are not alone. I pray your badges become a testament of your faith and a story of your perseverance. May you look upon your less-than-ideal badges on your sash and see the conqueror you are.

ABOUT THE AUTHOR

Evana is a God-fearing wife and mother of two children. She has become an expert at driving to appointments, crock-pot cooking, and managing piles of laundry. Evana loves her work as a pediatric speech-language pathologist, which allows her to help children with delays and disabilities. In the little bit of spare time she has left, she enjoys reading and writing. Her writing has appeared on sites like The Mighty, Key Ministry, and Scary Mommy. She contributed to Key Ministry's devotional books, *Spring Devotions for Special-Needs Families* and *Summer Devotions for Special-Needs Families*, which are both available from Amazon.

For more of her family's story, you can visit her blog, A Special Purposed Life, at http://specialpurposedlife.blogspot.com/.

www.ingramcontent.com/pod-product-compliance
Lightning Source LLC
Chambersburg PA
CBHW031300250726
48655CB00005B/2284